WORLDS OF HEALTH

WORLDS OF HEALTH
Exploring the Health Choices
of British Asian Mothers

Kate Reed

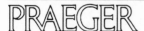

Westport, Connecticut
London

Library of Congress Cataloging-in-Publication Data

Reed, Kate, 1972–
    Worlds of health : exploring the health choices of British Asian Mothers /
by Kate Reed.
        p. cm.
    Includes bibliographical references and index.
    ISBN 0–89789–914–8 (alk. paper)
        1. Minority women—Health and hygiene—England—Leicester.
    2. South Asians—Health and hygiene—England—Leicester.   3.
    Mothers—Health and hygiene—England—Leicester.   4. Transcultural
    medical care—England—Leicester.   5. Health behavior—England—
    Leicester.   I. Title.
    RA564.86.R44   2003
    362.1'9089'95042542—dc21   2002033392

British Library Cataloguing in Publication Data is available.

Library of Congress Catalog Card Number: 2002033392
ISBN: 0–89789–914–8

First published in 2003

Praeger Publishers, 88 Post Road West, Westport, CT 06881
An imprint of Greenwood Publishing Group, Inc.
www.praeger.com

Printed in the United States of America

The paper used in this book complies with the
Permanent Paper Standard issued by the National
Information Standards Organization (Z39.48–1984).

10 9 8 7 6 5 4 3 2 1

To Mum, Dad, and Leo

Contents

Preface

Interest in ethnicity and identity has been far reaching over the last few decades. In particular there has been a significant amount of interest in the identities of children born to migrant parents. Studies on race and ethnicity during the 1970s that focused on young British-born ethnic minorities often saw them as neither wholly part of "home" or "host" culture, but rather as caught somewhere in between. In recent years studies have attempted to move away from static forms of categorization. The identities of British- or American-born minority ethnic groups are now seen as more fluid and multiply located, as something more complex and dynamic. In particular, explorations of the identity of such groups have often been seen as "hybrid," "syncretic," or "hyphenated," as combinational and transformative. While the identity of such a generation has become a prominent area of theory and research, the ways in which such syncretic identity affects more substantive concerns such as health has remained largely unexplored. This book aims to try to explore the links between ethnicity, identity, and health choices. It uses theoretical developments within the area of ethnicity and identity to explore substantive concerns.

The book started its life as a Ph.D. research project. In the initial research proposal I was keen to find out just how people's gendered, generational, and ethnic positioning affected health choices. What other factors were at play here? How influential were people's domestic situations, work environments, and so on? Behind this I also wanted to see how such choices were affected by the process of globalization. We live in a highly globalized world in which all kinds of products and services are available across national borders. Debates on globalization, though, have mostly stayed at the level of abstract theory. I wanted to go beyond this to look at how globalization affected individual people. I wanted to ask how globalization affected people's choices and use of health products and services.

The book is based on a study that focused on interviews with thirty British Asian women in the Midlands city of Leicester, United Kingdom. One might ask why I focused on British Asian women. This question is especially pertinent, as I am white and we are now living in an era where it seems only insider research (whatever that is) is viable. Why didn't I choose a different sample of the population? The reasons for focusing on South Asian women are numerous. In trying to look at the impact of globalization I wanted to explore the health choices of a widely globally dispersed migrant population, which the South Asian diaspora are. I also wanted to focus on a population with a history of nonbiomedical health systems. Ayurveda and Unani are, respectively, Hindu and Muslim medical systems originating in India. I wanted to look at how available these systems had become in the United Kingdom through migration. I also wanted to explore how much they were used by South Asians living in Britain. The reasons were also slightly more personal. Despite being white, I grew up in Leicester, which has a high South Asian population, and I had close connections with the South Asian population there. I had also used health care while visiting India. It was this encounter with Indian health care that provoked my desire to explore the use of various types of Indian medicine and remedies within the United Kingdom. In exploring South Asian women's health choices I have tried hard not to suggest the women involved in the research are a homogenous group in any way.

Through detailed accounts from the women in the study this book explores the ways in which ethnicity, gender, generation, and globalization affected the health choices of the women involved. It cannot, however, fully capture the warmth and humor of the women, nor the good times I had during that fieldwork. Indeed, my own health choices were substantially broadened throughout the research. I still think about and use Sakeena's remedies for a good complexion. A jar of Tiger Balm in my bathroom cabinet is a constant reminder of my interview with Samina. I still ponder Muskrat's offer to get me married.

On that note, I want to take this opportunity to thank the many people who have been involved with the production of this book in some way. In particular, I would like to thank all the women involved in the study. Thanks to Charlotte, Deepika, Gurinder, Harpreet, Inder, Jaipreet, Jameela, Jaya, Kishwar, Lata, Rambha, Maya, Mira, Muskrat, Nandita, Niru, Pavani, Priya, Ramila, Raminder, Reema, Rohini, Roopinder, Sakeena, Samina, Seema, Shahnaz, Sita, Surinder, and Zarhira. I would also like to thank the various community centers that helped me get started, including the Evington playgroup, East–West Centre, Bhagini Centre, Sikh Community Centre, and Sharma Women's Centre. Thanks are also due to the Faculty of Social Sciences, University of Southampton, for funding the project.

I would like to thank those in the department of Sociology and Social Policy at the University of Southampton, where the initial study took place; in particular, Graham Crow for the invaluable comments and support he gave throughout the project. I would also like to thank Waltraud Ernst, Susan Halford, and Bernard Harris, who were involved with the book in various ways and at differing stages. I would also like to thank my Ph.D. examiners, Professor Ursula Sharma and Dr. Caroline Knowles, for their insightful comments.

I would also like to thank Southampton friends (both old and new) Clare Alexander, Wendy Bottero, Derek McGhee, Traute Meyer, and Paul Sweetman. Thanks to Glyn Evans and Doreen Davis for all their help, support, and friendship. I would also like to thank those at the School of Social Policy,

Sociology, and Social Research, University of Kent at Canterbury, where the book was completed. In particular, thanks to Mary Evans, John Jervis, and Miri Song for support and encouragement. Clare Ungerson also deserves a mention here for always being so encouraging, both at Southampton and in Kent.

I would especially like to thank the people I love, my close friends and family. In particular, my partner in crime Melanie Semple for laughter, fun, and welcome dancing breaks. Thanks to others who became close to me at particular times during the four years of this project. Finally, special thanks to my family—my mum Ann, dad Lewis, siblings Sarah, Nick, and Dominic—for such love and support. I couldn't have done any of it without you.

Chapter 1

Introduction

This book is about the choices people make about their health, and what factors influence health choices. More specifically, the book explores the influence of ethnicity, gender, and generation on the health choices of British Asian mothers in a global era. The quest for both Western and non-Western health goods can readily be met in this age of globalization and migration. Western and non-Western products and services are widely available in both the local and global marketplaces. Faced by such choice and availability, we find ourselves free to draw "syncretically" on all kinds of health products and services; that is, to use a "mix and match" of such products and services. But what constitutes and constrains such syncrecy? How do ethnicity, gender, and generation affect access and use of a plurality of health goods and systems?

Existing studies that focus on the influence of ethnicity on health choices have been few and far between (Ahmad 1993). This is one significant factor that has led to the failure to provide culturally sensitive health services within the United Kingdom. Previous research has been characterized by large-scale epidemiological studies, which tend to have a clinical focus. Such research has focused on establishing patterns and explanations for the high rates of disease, such as diabetes, heart disease, hypertension, and so on, among ethnic minorities in the West (Ahmad 1996). These studies have not talked to real people about the choices they make about their health, nor about what might influence these choices.

The full impact of gender on the health choices of ethnic minority groups has yet to be explored. Black and Asian women have remained peripheral within the literature on health and have remained here as elsewhere objects of the biomedical Western gaze (Bayne-Smith 1996). There have been only a small number of studies that have focused specifically on the health choices of Black and Asian women (Thorogood 1990). In looking at the health of ethnic minority groups, studies have also often taken an ethnically reductive approach. Through this approach ethnic minorities have tended to be lumped together and treated as one category (Goldberg 1993). Even when the diversity of ethnic groups is recognized, studies have failed to take into account generational and immigration status. First, second, and third generations have been situated together. The emphasis tends to be on those who have migrated to the West, not on the unique position of those who were born and raised in the West.

We now live in an era characterized by a powerful phase of globalization (Massey 1994). Such a time includes an intensification of time–space compression, the opening up of possibilities on the global market through the global mediascape, and transcultural flows of goods and people. Boundaries in these circumstances dissolve and are crossed by everything from investment flows, to cultural influences, to satellite networks. This includes movement and widening accessibility of health products across the globe. Such an intense shift to the global is at the same time in tension with moves back to local placebound traditions. Globalization is characterized by the interplay between these local and global processes (Friedman 1994). While studies on identity have begun to explore the impact of these two-way processes on British-born migrants with both local and global ties, health research on ethnic minorities has yet to do so (Annandale 1998).

Departing from previous studies, this book explores the influence of ethnicity, gender, and generation on health choices. It moves away from deterministic models of ethnicity and health and situates health choices within the wider context of globalization. It focuses on the health choices of British Asian mothers; that is, Asian women who have either been born or lived in Britain from the age of five. By "health choice" I am referring here to our preferences and use of certain types of remedies and medicines. This book addresses issues of ethnicity and health, women's health, alternative health, generation, and identity, all within the context of globalization. Throughout the book two key questions are asked: First, are the health choices of British Asian mothers, women with both local and global connections, syncretic? Second, what social and cultural circumstances lie behind these health choices? This chapter outlines the significance of ethnicity, gender, and generation to health research. In exploring these key variables it states a need to develop a more fluid, globally located, and context-specific approach than has been used in previous studies. The chapter establishes such a theoretical framework. It also outlines the method used and geographically locates the study on which this book is based. The final section provides an outline of the book.

THE RACIALIZATION OF HEALTH

Within Britain, Ahmad (1993) argues, there have been two main trends regarding existing research on the health of minority ethnic groups. The first trend is a culturalist approach, the second is value-free epidemiology. The culturalist approach constructs and explains realities in terms of cultural differences, differences that are then usually equated with deviance and pathology. In this view any existing inequalities in health and access to health care are explained as resulting from cultural differences and deficits. Integration on the part of ethnic minority communities and cultural understanding and sensitivity on the part of health professionals then become the obvious solution; personal and institutional racism have no part in this equation.

An example of such could be seen during the influx of Black and Asian immigrants to Britain during the 1950s and 1960s (Ahmad 1993). During that time there was an overall increase in the rate of TB among the general population. This increase was blamed on the new immigrants, and TB became known as an immigrant disease. Immigrant groups were labelled as problematic and as breeders of ill health. These types of culturalist approaches to research have led to culturalist health policy. An example of this is the stop rickets campaign (Rocheron 1988). Rickets, once a common problem among White children, was acknowledged as a disease of poverty that was controlled through fortifying margarine with vitamin D, improvements in standard of living and nutrition, and universally available free milk to schools. With the knowledge of a higher prevalence among Asian children in the 1970s it emerged as an Asian disease signified by a new name, "Asian rickets." Rather than seeing rickets as a product of poor conditions migrants faced on arrival in Britain, it was explained in terms of non-British eating and living habits and perhaps a genetic deficiency in absorbing vitamins into the bloodstream or in synthesizing sunlight. The predicted long-term answer to Asian rickets was seen to lie in education and in a change to Western diet and lifestyle. This was reflected in the official response of the Department of Health and Social Security (DHSS) working party and the resulting stop rickets campaign.

Ahmad (1993) argues that the second trend within health research on ethnic minority group health has been a supposedly value-free epidemiology, using the notion of a disinterested value-free scientific observer who makes pronouncements on the basis of carefully collected evidence that uses a rigorous scientific method, usually clinical questionnaires. Such studies focus on establishing and explaining patterns for the high rates of disease among minorities (Pitchumon and Saran 1976). According to Lambert and Sevak (1996) these epidemiological studies have demonstrated an increased incidence of conditions such as diabetes and heart disease in the groups under study relative to the White population, rather than, for example, as a result of expressed concerns emanating from within these groups. As Eade (1997) argues, such studies focus on quantitative data and biomedical models of disease. Views are sought only from the professional structure of health provision. The health choices of ordinary people do not inform the debates, nor does non-Western medicine. According to Ahmad (1993) these trends often involve a racialization of health research. They assume that populations can be divided only into ethnic or racial groups, taking these groups as primary categories and using these categories for explanatory purposes. Stratification by class, income, gender, and so on are seen as relatively unimportant. Ill health is depoliticized and individualized, and the afflicted are treated in isolation from their social, economic, and citizenship contexts. This in turn legitimates existing inequalities and maintains the status quo.

One of the main aims of this book is to follow calls by Ahmad (1993) and others for the sociology of health and illness to recognize ethnicity as an important (but not the only) sociological dimension and to incorporate it into explanations of health-based choices. As this book will show, ethnicity and culture are important parts of a complex web of influences on health choices, which includes a range of influences from family to geographical location. Throughout the book culture is defined as a set of beliefs and ideas that a group draws on to identify and manage the problems of their everyday lives. It is a dynamic entity that changes to incorporate fresh ideas and perspectives as people develop new ways of responding to their environments. This moves away from approaches that see culture as predicting precisely in a positivist way what people believe and how they will behave (Kelleher 1996). The term "ethnicity," a historically contested term, has been used to describe groups with shared language, religion, or nationality, but the idea of shared culture has perhaps been the most crucial issue. The term is used here generally to refer to the sense of belonging to a community that may not necessarily be defined in racial terms (Bradley 1996). I have left the definition of ethnicity deliberately open in order to move away from deterministic approaches that draw rigid lines around social groupings.

INVISIBLE WOMEN:
GENDER, ETHNICITY, AND HEALTH

Over recent years there has been a significant body of feminist writing surrounding the area of women's health. Within sociology, White feminists have provided valuable and challenging research literature on gender in relation to, among other areas, caring for the sick, the medicalization process, nursing, mothering, the sexist nature of medical ideology and institutional structures, and positivist methods. Research has highlighted the omission of women from large-scale epidemiological studies. Doyal (1995) has demonstrated that research on conditions such as heart disease and cancer traditionally uses only men as study participants. Bayne-Smith (1996) argues, therefore, that when women are prescribed highly toxic medications on the basis of research done solely on men, women are in essence placed in jeopardy by the medical establishment. Kirchstein (1991) suggests that biomedical research continues to reflect the bias of White men. The focus regarding women's health tends to be on women's reproductive capacities; little research has focused on non-reproductive-related conditions that affect women, such as osteoporosis or incontinence. Doyal has also pointed out that while women are well represented within the health care professions they are overrepresented within the low-paid professions. A number of studies in the United Kingdom have also found that women's own assessment of their health continues to be consistently worse then that of men (Blaxter 1990).

Even though research on women's health in general has begun to move into the mainstream, there continues to be grossly inadequate information about the health status and choice of women of color. White feminists within sociology, despite valuable research within all the areas mentioned here, are guilty of excluding women from ethnic minorities (Ahmad 1993). Black women were nowhere to be found in the earlier work of leading British feminist writers like Oakley (1980). There are only a small number of studies that look at the choices of Black and Asian women (Thorogood 1990). These studies are useful in that they look at the health choices of ethnic minority groups. They have tended to find mixed results: some women favoring non-Western health remedies, others favoring Western. Within these studies, health choices are analyzed within the context of ethnicity alongside reference to women's social circumstances. This book contributes to and expands on the focus of these studies. It does so by demonstrating a broader link between health choice, ethnicity, gender, and globalization.

A prominent area of research regarding White women's health has been women's activities as caregivers, in families and in society at large, and as primary consumers of health care for themselves and others (Graham 1984, 1993; Miles 1991). Women urge their loved ones to seek medical care, they make the doctor appointments for their family members, and they purchase and replenish over-the-counter medicines for the family's bathroom cabinet. Similarly, they are more likely than men to monitor the health status of extended family members, to become caretakers of the elderly and infirm, and to be the ones to leave work to look after sick children (Graham 1993). While there have been a number of studies in Britain that have highlighted the role of working-class mothers in mediating the health of other members of the family and the importance of their health beliefs in shaping family health behaviors (Blaxter 1990; Cornwell 1984), little research has focused on the health choices of ethnic minority mothers. Bowes and Domokos (1993) point out the importance of looking at mothers when looking at health. In their research on Punjabi Muslim women in Glasgow they found that women are still largely responsible for the health of their partners and children and other relations.

This book situates women's health in a wider social context. It turns the epidemiological approach on its head. It aims to understand social relations along the lines of race and gender, along with the social construction of health and illness, offering important examples of how such links are forged in concrete situations. This book takes up the focus on women's use of a variety of medicines by existing studies such as Donovan's (1986) research on South Asian and Afro-Caribbean women and Bowes and Domokos's (1993) research on South Asian women. In particular, this book picks up on the findings of previous studies that focused on the role of women as mediators of family health (Blaxter and Paterson 1982). Drawing on the findings of an empirical study, this book explores women's health choices by focusing on their position as mediators of family health. The study focused on mothers in order to gain information not just about women's health choices, but also those of children and other family members. By doing this, women's gendered and generational positions within the family are explored.

THE SIGNIFICANCE OF GENERATION

In most studies on ethnicity and health, generations and minorities have tended to be grouped together in an ethnically reductive approach (Goldberg 1993). Studies that have explored differences between generations have often focused on epidemiological differences. For instance, Greenslade, Madden, and Pearson (1997), in their research on Irish migrants to the United Kingdom, show differences in patterns of health among first- and second-generation migrants and those between northern and southern Irish. Similarly, Marks and Hilder (1997), in their research on European Jewish immigrants and Bengali immigrants in East London, show how patterns of health change over the period of settlement and so vary dramatically over generations. Little work has been conducted that looks at the differences and similarities in health choices between generations. Researchers have often alluded to the differences between generations in this context but failed to explore them. Kraut (1997), in his paper on Italian migrants, looks at the differences in the use of modern and traditional beliefs among Italian immigrants to the United States from the turn of the century onward. He found that, although the use of traditional remedies such as the "evil eye" was still prevalent at times among all generations of Italian migrants, there tended to be a greater use of modern remedies among second- and third-generation migrants and a greater use of traditional medicine among older generations.

This book focuses on the generation of South Asians born or living in Britain in 1998 from the age of five. It takes up some of the ideas put forward by writers on identity (e.g., Parker 1995), who have focused on the unique identity of diaspora members born to a Western society. Earlier studies on children of postwar migrants during the 1970s identified this generation as caught between two cultures (Watson 1977). The "problem" was that they might not integrate smoothly into British society; the authoritarian and old-fashioned cultures of their parents were deemed to be holding them back (Parker 1995). In recent years studies on ethnicity and identity have moved away from such approaches to explore the syncretic, multiply located, and changing identity of this particular generation. As Annandale (1998) argues, writers on ethnicity and health have yet to take this up. Similarly, within the United States there has been a proliferation of writing on issues of identity concerning second-generation American Asians (Rocher 1994). American Asians have been compared with British Asians within this literature. For instance, Mukhi (1996) makes comparisons between American and British Asians. She talks of a transnational community of what she terms "hyphenated Indians." She argues that the hyphenated American Indian is heavily influenced by British South Asians as well as by India itself. She draws on the complexity of colonial and postcolonial landscapes to present her argument of the transnational hyphenated Indian.

Kelleher (1996), in his work on ethnicity and health, recognizes the difficulties faced by certain ethnic minority groups born in English society. He argues that although the parents of these groups migrated to England they themselves were born and educated in the United Kingdom. They have had close contact with "English" culture. He goes on to argue that there are grounds for including them as members of the parent group. However, it may be that this membership is less central to their identity because they have moved out of that association with the parental generation as a result of education and socioeconomic change. As yet, however, research has failed to put this group at the center of research on ethnicity and health to explore the ideas of syncrecy and hybridity and to look at how important ethnicity is within this group's health choices. Within this book the impact of generation on health choice is seen as an important variable. In particular, the generational position of British-born South Asian migrants is explored. The term "South Asian" refers in this context to people from India, Pakistan, Bangladesh, and Sri Lanka. This also includes those migrating to Britain from South Asia via East Africa (Ballard 1994). The terms "British South Asian" and "British Asian" are used within the context of this book to refer to those of South Asian parentage who were born and/or raised within Britain.

MIXING REMEDIES:
THE CONFLICTS OF PAST RESEARCH

Existing studies on the health choices of ethnic minority groups have tended to find various patterns regarding the use of Western and non-Western medicine. In her research on Afro-Caribbean and Asian women in London, Donovan (1986) found mixed results. In Donovan's study, while Afro-Caribbean women used a plurality of medicines, Asian women used mostly Western medicines. Armstrong and Pierce (1996), on the other hand, in their research on diabetes among Afro-Caribbeans in London, found no mention of folk remedies, which they argued was different from the Asian experience. Eade (1997), in his research on Bangladeshi communities in Tower Hamlets, London, argues that minorities and migrants draw on a plurality of medicines, combining both non-Western and Western. He suggests that this drawing on a number of discourses is a part of the dynamic and contested process of cultural construction as immigrants adapt to the conditions of urban life within the West. Eade's approach is useful within the context of this book. With an emphasis on dynamic and contested construction of health choices it enables us to move beyond temporally static approaches and approaches that locate health choices within one type of medicine.

The question over use of different types of remedies, however, becomes more complex when we consider whether Western and non-Western medical systems can be seen as completely distinct. Brady, Kunitz, and Nash (1997) argue that we should not look at these systems separately, setting Western and non-Western medicine up against one another as binary oppositions. In their research on aboriginal health, they argue that non-Western medicine is often set up as antithetical to the Cartesian dualist model of Western biomedicine. They suggest that the Western medical model of health is not quite as monolithic as it is portrayed. Brady, Kunitz, and Nash suggest that there is, after all, a long history of acceptance in the West of the relationship between affective and physical states and the influence of the mind on illness being expressed in different ways in different countries. They argue that non-Western medicine, which in their research takes the form of aboriginal medicine, embraces concepts of health that are practical in ways that on occasions belie more romantic conceptualizations. There is, therefore, a false dichotomy in presenting Western and non-Western medical systems as polar opposites. Within the context of this study it was more fruitful to explore whether the women within the research themselves distinguished between discrete and separate systems or saw crossovers.

Exploring the relationships between systems themselves brings me around to the issue of what constitutes "non-Western" medicine within this book. Ideas about what constitutes alternative, indigenous, non-Western, unorthodox, or nonconventional medicine remains a contested domain. All the terms suffer from the same problems. All set Western medicine up as the "normal" and anything else as abnormal or fringe, as "other." In light of this, the term chosen was "non-Western" medicine or remedies. While the term "non-Western" is as problematic in some respects as any of the other terms, it is used with caution. Within the book it is recognized that not all alternative medicine is non-Western. In looking at South Asian women, however, the book is mostly concerned with those systems originating from non-Western contexts.

The following two sections on syncrecy and context provide the general theoretical framework that informs each chapter of this book. This framework was chosen because it provides the greatest explanatory power to understand the intersections of ethnicity, gender, generation, and globalization on health choices. It enables an analysis that can understand the dynamic, diverse, and changing influences on women's health choices. The framework is established here so that each chapter can work through each subtle shade of its practice in relation to each different formation of illness, family, religion, community, space, and location.

EXPLORING SYNCRETIC HEALTH CHOICES

The idea that health choices are syncretic plays on the complex interweaving of ethnicity, culture, and material circumstance for this generational group. Syncrecy here refers to the mixing and matching of different types of health remedies and medicines. It does not suggest a complete collapse between medical systems, but rather refers to the creation of new combinations of medicines in health choice. It is used to explore the idea that the women in the study draw their health choices from a combination of non-Western and Western medicine.

Authors such as Clifford (1997) and Gilroy (1993) have begun to explore the tensions between continuity, fracturing, commonality, and difference that are present in all forms of identity. Gilroy (1993), in talking about the Black diaspora in both America and Britain, describes a cultural formation that has arisen from the diaspora, which he names the "Black Atlantic" to convey the idea that it is a hybrid, a mix of elements from Western culture (both British and American), from the Caribbean, and from the homelands of African slaves. Just as capitalism was founded on trade between these locations, culture is shaped by journeys (actual and symbolic) between the areas. Gilroy uses the idea to attack the ideal of the recovery of a "lost" or "original" African culture. The notion of hybridity has been developed by Bhabha (1992) to describe contemporary ethnic identity. For example, Indian people settled in Britain are affected by aspects of both, or all, the cultures to which they are exposed. They are not simply British or stuck "between two cultures," as Watson (1977) would argue, but rather draw on a "hyphenated" or syncretic identity, which is different from an Indian or Chinese person who has never left Asia.

The concepts of syncrecy and syncretism have also been used in some research on health. Fitzpatrick (1984) uses the concept of syncrecy in terms of general lay views about health. He argues that lay views are syncretic in origin in that they originate from distinct and disparate sources and are continually being reworked in the light of experience. The term has also been used to explore medical systems themselves. Leslie (1992) suggests that medical systems are syncretic, incorporating into their centers a mix and match of different systems. However, as Annandale (1998) notes, while there has been an exploration of global diaspora and the emergence of syncretic cultures within identity studies, and separately the use of the concept of syncrecy in studies on health, to date there has been little attempt to draw on frameworks of syncrecy when exploring ethnicity and identity within the context of health. This book develops those frameworks within a health context.

One must use current theoretical buzzwords such as syncrecy or hybridity with caution, particularly in regard to race and ethnicity. Narayan (1996) argues that anthropologists are well advised to discard an emphasis on pristine authenticity, taking heed of hybridity, innovation, and global connections. However, as Parker (1995) argues, both syncrecy and hybridity are uneasy biologistic metaphors for combination, which can connote a state rather than a process, and could lead to a position that implies a pure origin and an alternative that when combined together produce a new term, "the hybrid." He argues the emphasis should instead be on process. Both terms run the risk of glorifying disjuncture, producing a new rigidity and an academic alterity that merely values itself for its own state. Grewal and Kaplan (1994) also argue that by suggesting in any way that diaspora are syncretic or hybrid one is in danger of setting up the White subject as somehow pure.

In order to avoid using syncrecy to denote a "state," some kind of purity or a reification of a "between two cultures" type approach, a fluid framework of syncrecy was developed within this study. The concept of syncrecy is used here to capture and explore crossovers and tensions between categories of difference. The term is taken to resist the complete collapse of categories of difference. While recognizing that at times there may be crossovers between categories, syncrecy also allows the potential for tensions between categories at particular times and contexts. In this sense, rather than being a fixed or static framework, syncrecy is seen rather as fluid and polyvocal. To echo Gilroy's (1993) argument, syncretic forms are never repeated in quite the same way, but are reworked and reinscribed differently in differing contexts. Syncrecy, then, is an analytical not a chronological framework, which will change according to historical, local, and personal context. Within this book the framework of syncrecy is used to look at the way in which West and non-West are seen as mixed, both locally and globally, in a reciprocal context. This is used to look at the tension for British Asian women between West and non-West. Such a framework of syncrecy enables the development of a suitable paradigm within which to look at the health choices of British Asian women.

Within this framework I move away from a view of health choices as fixed in time. Current writers on identity make explicit the argument that identities are fluid and complex. Indeed, those writing from a postmodern perspective argue that the postmodern subject has no fixed identity; the unified, completed, secure, and coherent identity is fantasy. Similarly, Radley and Billig (1996) argue that health beliefs should not been seen as static but as processual as people actively construct their identities. Within this book I will suggest that health choices cannot be constructed as single narratives, but change according to time and context.

LOCALIZING THE GLOBAL: HEALTH CHOICES IN CONTEXT

In discussing utilizing postmodern approaches from studies on identity and ethnicity within a health context, Annandale (1998) urges caution. She argues that on the one hand we might see the more fluid approach to identity as the ultimate "way out" of the problems that have arisen when an individual's health status or health choices are rather uncritically read off their designated ethnic group status (in both qualitative and quantitative research). On the other hand, she argues that concern has been expressed that euphemisms of diversity can act as a smoke screen for the entrenchment of inequality (Smith 1993). While some imply that more fluid identities are a product of global social change, particularly in the European context, others warn that such approaches are themselves Areocentric and deeply racialized, as they generate a "vision which renders the immiserated irrelevant and blacks, in particular, as ornaments without agency or resistance" (Harris 1993, 35). In order to avoid the relativism of such approaches and the reification of culturalist approaches to health outlined earlier, the framework of syncrecy is also explored through the influence of respondents' contextual circumstances. By "context" I mean a broad range of circumstances within respondents' lives that are not just about their ethnic or generational positions. This book includes circumstances that range from familial, to material socioeconomic, to wider structural constraints.

Previous research on ethnicity and health choice has tended to view ethnicity as the only or, at the very least, the primary factor in determining health choices. As Bowes and

Domokos (1993) argue, much research has focused on culture as a causative factor. They argue that this leads investigators to ignore influences on health choices such as socioeconomic group, housing conditions, and access to health care. As argued earlier, this has filtered down to a culture-blaming approach in health policy (Ahmad 1993). It is important to look at factors other than culture. Nagel (1994) develops the term "symbolic ethnicity" to look at how factors other than ethnicity affect people's life choices. Symbolic ethnicity is characterized as a nostalgic allegiance to the culture of the immigrant generation. However, this allegiance is "symbolic" in the sense that other factors such as work and class heavily inform identity and daily practice.

As well as exploring the influence of culture and ethnicity, this book focuses on the importance of factors, such as the significance of women's access to health services, work, other material circumstances, and location in time and space in influencing health choices. In recognizing how factors other than culture affect health behavior, Ahmad (1996) gives the example of different experiences of childbirth in Pakistan. One woman's experience of child birth involved the use of an obstetrician, a second involved the use of a Dai (traditional birth attendant without any biomedical training, adhering to a forty-day recuperation process of Chilla), and the third worked in road construction before and after birth. All three were Muslim women employed in present-day Pakistan, but their lives were differentiated by class, urban–rural divisions, and access to health care. All three types of childbirth are part of Pakistani culture and tradition regarding pregnancy and childbirth.

While acknowledging that health choices are shaped by more than ethnic and cultural processes, however, one should be careful not to move to a position that is overly deterministic. To take the position that health choices are completely determined by external forces leads to an approach that denies agency. It also tends to ignore the influence of other factors on health choices; for example, the influence of the family. This is why such a broad definition of contextual circumstances is drawn upon, to incorporate personal, social, and structural influences. This avoids a complete denial of agency and influences relating not just to external factors. It is important to recognize that groups may use non-Western health care. For instance, Kelleher and Islam (1996) carried out research on the incidence of diabetes among Bangladeshis in the United Kingdom. They found that people mixed both Western and non-Western health discourses when managing diabetes on a daily level. On the whole they saw diabetes as a problem that had to be managed by Western medicine, and did not appear to think folk remedies had much to offer them apart from widely used karella (a bitter vegetable). Some said that they had been told by the doctor to use karella and one person claimed that it was on a hospital diet sheet, which is an interesting example of Western doctors being prepared to work with lay ideas.

Kelleher and Islam's (1996) study demonstrates the complex nature of choices about health care and how a number of factors are taken into account when choosing remedies and healthcare. From the findings of the study they suggested that their respondents were not simply making personal choices about what to eat. Through integrating their traditional foods with other internationally available foods like rice crispies, fish fingers, and so on, their respondents were confronted by the dialectic of the local and the global. Alongside this, respondent's traditional ways of thinking about life and death were also being challenged by a medical treatment predicated on a notion of risk reduction (Kelleher and Islam 1996). All their respondents within the constraints of their situations were actively constructing their lives as people with diabetes, and their cultural beliefs were one of the resources they used. The frameworks, the structures of relevance that they drew on were shared, but individuals constructed their own lives within them.

This exploration of both syncrecy and context within women's health choices is held in tension throughout this book through a dialectical approach. While not entirely polarized, nor are the syncretic and the contextual wholly joined. A dialectical approach enables us to ground the two theories of syncrecy and context and provides a wider framework throughout the book particularly when focusing on the operationalization of research categories. Schrijvers's (1993) notion of dialectic will be used here. She defines dialectic as a reflexive approach that makes room for a plurality of views and multivocal discourse. In this approach knowledge is seen as an outcome of dialogues of inter- and intrasubjective communications and of the confrontations of differing images of reality. Knowledge in this way is seen as a temporary construct, determined historically, locally, and personally. In allowing for plurality and multivocal discourse encapsulated in tension, this approach moves us beyond a theoretical framework based on static hierarchical binaries. It enables an exploration of both global and local processes, and recognizes the importance of history, context, and experiential rooting.

METHODOLOGY

The main purpose of this book is to explore the influence of ethnicity, gender, and generation on the health choices of British Asian mothers in a global era. The book is based on interviews with thirty British Asian mothers in Leicester conducted in the late 1990s. The British Asian women within the study adhered to various religions, they came from a range of social classes, and their ages ranged from early twenties to early forties. They all had at least one child of school age. Blaxter and Paterson (1982) highlight the important role of women as mediators of family health. The decision to focus on mothers arose out of this for the purpose of finding out not just about the women's health choices regarding themselves but also about the health choices of their family members. While the respondents were made up of a heterogeneous set of people, it should be recognized that such a sample is not representative. The claims made about health choices outlined within this book are specific to this particular group of women. However, while we cannot generalize from this sample of thirty British Asian mothers, the study does offer a base from which comparisons with women in other positions and contexts can be explored. In order to access respondents, I approached playgroups, community groups, and women's centers. The women within these groups and centers were keen to be involved.

In order to explore women's attitudes to health and to access health choices and the meanings women attach to them, a method was needed that generated "open" data rather than imposing a formalized set of questions (Oakley 1981). The method chosen to access this type of material was in-depth semistructured interviews. Within the research, while I used an interview schedule that included a focus on women's general health, their experience of specific illness, and their social context and identity, this was flexible and women were free to talk about the things they felt most pertinent. Drawing on Radley and Billig's (1996) work, women's accounts on health were viewed as more than just the women's views on health and illness; rather, they were viewed as part of the ongoing construction of their identity. By giving detailed accounts of their health and illness, women disclosed information about the fluid locations they occupy and how these vary according to time and context (Popay and Groves 2000). This allowed me to access the ways in which women saw their social circumstances, ethnicity, gender, and generation as influencing their health over time.

Prior to the main body of interviews, an informal pilot discussion group was conducted in order to refine the interview schedule. This involved four women from a community playgroup, all of whom had small children. All interviews from the research were transcribed and from these transcripts themes were developed. The interviews have remained confidential and the names of the women involved have been changed.

In conducting the fieldwork, there was one major methodological concern related to the issue of race. How could I, a White researcher, interview Asian women? Rhodes (1994) and others have raised questions surrounding the issue of a White researcher undertaking research with non-White respondents. As Back (1993) argues, in Britain the central issue within the debate on research practice in the sociology of race has been the ability of the White researcher to understand and empathize with Black experiences of racism. Ram (1996) argues that to do such research is difficult and that to hold a similar structural position to respondents is particularly beneficial in gaining information. However, as Kelleher (1996) suggests, while there are good reasons for Black researchers to research Black communities (one reason being that they might be better able to gain both physical and psychological access to people), interviewing across race can work. It may sometimes even have benefits, such as people being able to talk more freely to community "outsiders." M. L. Anderson (1993) notes from his own research across race that White scholars can develop and utilize tensions in their own identities to enable them to see different aspects of minority group experiences and beliefs.

With this in mind, the methodological approach adopted throughout this study is a "feminist" perspective based on the idea of "partial identity" (Haraway 1988; Harding 1991). The benefit of the partial perspective is that it recognizes both differences and similarities in women's experiences. While there are differences in experience, positioning, and power relations between women, there are also commonalities. We can "partially identify" with other women through our various experiences. For example, in the context of research, while we may be of a different race to respondents, we may be in the same socioeconomic group and share experience there. These tensions and commonalities can help to build rapport within a research situation while acknowledging women's differing experiences. In adopting this perspective a level of caution must also be applied. The partial identity framework has been critiqued for its evasion of research responsibility. Haraway (1988) argues that researchers feign commonality when it suits and emphasize diversity if issues of responsibility come to the fore. It is important to keep this in mind when recognizing both commonalities and differences between researcher and researched. In taking this approach the study is also based on a politics of location that acknowledges people's individual social circumstances.

LOCATING THE PROJECT

The research on which this book is based was conducted in Leicester for two reasons. First, Leicester has a significant South Asian population of varying religions and socioeconomic classes. Second, previous research on ethnic minority health choices has focused on carrying out research in areas such as London or Glasgow; few studies on minority health have been carried out in the Midlands, which is surprising because of the area's significant Asian population. Leicester was chosen partly to see what differences there might be from previous studies relating to geographical location.

Leicester is known historically as a booming industrial city, famous for its hosiery, knitwear, and footwear manufacturing, and more recently for engineering, printing, adhesive manufacturing, and food processing. By the mid-1960s Leicester was at the height of the boom. During this time it became a magnet town for immigrants from the Indian subcontinent, the Caribbean, and, by the later 1960s, East and Central Africa. According to data from the 1991 census (Leicester City Council 1991b), Leicester ranks fifth in terms of absolute numbers of all ethnic minorities, second for all Asian groups, first for people of Indian origin, but only thirty-fifth for those who classify themselves as Black. However, outside the London area it is the local authority with the highest percentage of all ethnic minorities. It has a White population of around 71.5 percent, a Black population of around 2.4 percent, an Asian population of 23.7 percent, and a Chinese and "other" ethnic population of 2.4 percent. While Leicester's Asian population includes Ugandan, Kenyan, Tanzanian, Punjabi, Pakistani/Bangladeshi, and those from the rest of the subcontinent (e.g., Gujarat), the population is now heavily weighted toward East African Asians and

Gujaratis, both Muslim and Hindu. (East African Asians are Asians who originated from the Indian subcontinent but then settled in East Africa.)

The single most important feature that makes Leicester different from other cities that experienced postwar migration is its East African connection. In the 1950s the immigrants came because of the push factor from those newly independent African countries intent on Africanizing their economies, a process that prompted the imposition of much tighter entry controls by successive British governments (Marett 1989). Leicester attracted East Africans, largely because of its laissez-faire policy to immigration. This stance was based on cautious pragmatism rather than on deliberate policies with regard to its immigrants. Many Asians moved to Leicester initially because of the prosperity, the low incidence of strikes, and the range of industries (including work for women). There were other reasons for migration to Leicester, ease of access to other cities being one of them. Situated in the middle of England, Leicester is at the focus of its communications networks, a very significant factor for minority groups who wish to visit and be visited by relatives and friends for personal, social, religious, and commercial reasons. Finally, there was cheap housing available (Marett 1989).

Leicester still has a growing South Asian population concentrated in Highfields, Melton Road, Belgrave Road, and Narborough Road. These are all inner-city areas: residential, business, and industrial, some in the prosperous area of Oadby. There are over forty clubs, societies, and organizations devoted to the social and welfare needs of Asian groups: There are three Hindu temples, three Sikh Gurwaras, and two Muslim mosques and an Islamic foundation (Marett 1989). There was also the opening of a Bollywood cinema by 1974 on Belgrave Road, "The Natraj." Jeffers, Hoggett, and Harrison (1996) argue that Leicester is made up of White and ethnic minority communities far less defensive than those in other localities, such as Tower Hamlets. Moreover, the East African community has, by virtue of the particular colonial role it had played in East African history, become partially anglicized and therefore found the transition to the United Kingdom easier than many other minorities elsewhere. These factors have made it an ideal location for gaining a sample. Also, because of Leicester's central location it is an ideal place in which to explore local–global links and the diverse and multifaceted nature of the South Asian diaspora.

OUTLINE

In exploring local and global influences on health choices this book marks a departure from previous studies on ethnicity and health, with their rigid and determinist conceptualizations. It offers a broader and more flexible approach. It addresses key questions on ethnicity, women's health, alternative health, identity, and globalization. The dynamic framework is one that takes into account the influence of globalization while also recognizing the significance of social context. Within this book, two key issues are explored: first, the idea that women's health choices are syncretic; second, the role and importance of contextual circumstances on women's health choices. These issues and their relationship to the women's position as British Asians (that is, women of a particular ethnic and generational group) with wider diasporic connections will be explored in detail.

Chapter 2 addresses what is relevant to us all: the conceptualization of health and illness. The chapter explores the ways in which the women's use of Western and non-Western health remedies relate to particular types of illness. Women tend to use non-Western medicine for general illnesses, such as colds, and Western medicine for serious illness, such as cancer. Choice of health remedies will also be related to the women's position as British Asians, as members of a globally dispersed ethnic group with access to a plurality of medicines across the globe.

Chapter 3 addresses the influence of family, generation, and the life course on health choices. Drawing on women's local, national, and global family ties, this chapter examines the ways in which family, generation, and life course affect British Asian women's use of Western and non-Western remedies. In particular, there has been significant interest in the literature on women's roles as mediators of family health. In capitalizing on this interest, Chapter 3 explores women's gendered positioning within the family. It explores their role as mothers and mediators of family health, and the ways in which they influence family use of syncretic remedies.

Chapter 4 examines three core concerns within disciplines such as anthropology and sociology: religion, community, and identity. First, the chapter explores the significance of religious ritual in the women's health accounts. Second, the chapter investigates the influence of community in all its varying forms, from religious to pan-Asian, on the use of both Western and non-Western remedies. Finally, the chapter places health within the context of wider debates on ethnicity and identity. The chapter looks at the ways in which respondents' syncretic position as British Asians both influences and reflects their use of syncretic remedies.

Chapter 5 asks what the influences are of geographical location, space, and globalization on the women's use of health remedies. In particular, this chapter highlights the significance of the women's membership in a globally dispersed ethnic group. The chapter first looks at the influence of the respondents' geographical location in Leicester, and then moves on to highlight the significance of respondents' connections and resources within South Asia. This will include explorations of women's health-product purchases and use of health care in South Asia and in other diasporic contexts. The chapter concludes by summing up the ways in which syncrecy is spatially located and opened up in both local and global contexts.

In the concluding chapter the main findings of this research are summarized, focusing on the ways in which respondents drew on different types of health remedies according to their contextual and material circumstances, from family through to geographical location. I highlight the significance of the women's position as British Asians (as women raised in Britain with membership in a globally dispersed ethnic group) in enabling women access to a plurality of Western and non-Western goods. The impact of migration alongside this intense phase of globalization highlights the increasing accessibility of a plurality of health products for certain groups in society. The implications of the findings in terms of research and policy are also explored.

Chapter 2

Concepts of Health
and Illness

This chapter addresses what is relevant to us all: the conceptualization of health and illness. We all define health and illness in certain ways and make certain decisions based on our experiences of health and illness. For instance, we all have ideas about when illness warrants a visit to the pharmacist or when to go and see the doctor. Our experiences of illness therefore significantly influence our health choices. Drawing on data from the broader study, this chapter explores the ways in which women's health choices relate to particular types of illness. This chapter shows how women are more likely to use non-Western remedies for general illnesses, such as colds and flu, while they draw almost solely on Western medicine for serious illness (e.g., from diabetes to cancer). This chapter explores the ways in which illness becomes categorized and dealt with in both the public and the domestic realm. In making these arguments, I will highlight the ways in which such categorization of illness intersects with women's locations in the life course and their position as British Asians. This will show that although illness can be seen to play an influential role in health choices, such influence must also be based in a temporal, social, and cultural context.

CONCEPTUALIZING HEALTH AND ILLNESS

There appears to be great diversity regarding definitions of health. The definition of health given by the World Health Organization rests on the idea of a total state of physical, mental, and social well-being (Spector 1996). This is situated in opposition to the medical model of health, which is based on the idea of the absence of disease (Jones 1994). Lay definitions offer more diversity still, as they are mediated through peoples social and cultural contexts. When lay people are actually asked what health is, many are unable clearly to define health and illness, although they can say readily enough whether they regard themselves as healthy or not (Blaxter 1990). To feel healthy or sick is a personal experience, but concepts of health and illness are learned by drawing on the accumulated knowledge of the relevant culture. In trying to account for the diversity in definitions of health, Jones (1994) suggests that "health is a state of being that is subject to wide individual, social and cultural interpretation; it is produced by the interplay of individual perceptions and social influences" (p. 3). This is a useful definition in that it allows for the interaction of a complex set of factors that may influence our definitions of health.

Whatever meaning is given to health by lay people, ill health represents a breakdown in the normal expected state of health and well-being, a deviation from how things should be when things go wrong. It is a transition from a normal phenomenological mode of bodily silence (Leder 1990) to bodily alienation or betrayal (S. J. Williams 1996, 2000).[1] Kleinman (1980) argues that illness refers to those human experiences that represent interpersonal and cultural reaction to symptoms or discomfort.

For the purposes of this book, Cornwell's (1984) tripartite categorization of illness proves particularly useful. She argues that when lay people think about illness they often situate illness within categories. She developed a tripartite system of categories of illness from information drawn from twenty-four respondents interviewed in a study in East London. She argues that her respondents' conceptualizations can be placed within three main categories of illness. "Normal" illness was what most people were expected to get sometimes, such as infectious diseases in childhood or colds and flu in winter. "Real" illness meant major disabling and life-threatening diseases. "Health problems" was the third category, those afflications that are not illness but are associated with natural processes, such as aging or the reproductive cycle, and also mental health problems, such as depression and anxiety. The category of health problems that cause pain, distress, and much suffering is especially important for women because it includes problems inherent in menstruation, childbirth, pregnancy, and menopause, and because they suffer far more (or at least are seen to suffer more) than men do from such conditions as depression, anxiety, and agoraphobia.

While we can roughly categorize illness within lay accounts in such a way, it is important to recognize that choices about health are specific to individual circumstances. The importance attached to possible courses of action differ from one individual to another according to his or her position in the social structure and prevalent social norms (Miles 1991). Guo (2000) argues that the type of behavior in dealing with illness is heavily influenced by sociocultural expectations and perceptions concerning illness. In this way categories of health and illness should not be seen as fixed, but must be seen as socially constructed notions that mean different things to different people in different times and contexts. There may be consensus as to fatal diseases being "real" illnesses, but how to deal with them is often a disputed matter among both lay and professionally trained people (Miles 1991).

In what follows I will focus on the respondents' use of syncretic remedies in relation to three categories of health and illness: normal illness, health problems, and real illness. While exploring the influence of illness on women's health choices, the influence of individual social context will also be accounted for. While the women's accounts about illnesses can be situated in illness categories, neither the categories nor the women's accounts should be completely fixed. Rather, they should be seen as temporally and contextually specific. In acknowledgment of this the influence of social context (for instance, geographical location and social networks) will be included in the analysis.

SYNCRETIZING "NORMAL" ILLNESS

Within Cornwell's (1984) tripartite classification system, people talked about certain general conditions that fall under the guise of normal illness. In her study, normal illness ranged from the infectious diseases of childhood, such as chicken pox and mumps, to adulthood infections of the kidneys, tonsils, and sinuses, as well as stomach problems, fevers, and some common respiratory diseases. Women within this study also grouped certain general illnesses together and had particular beliefs about them and behaved accordingly. Illness that fell under the guise of normal illness for the women were much the same as those described in Cornwell's (1984) study, including colds, fevers, and flu.

Studies focusing on lay health choices demonstrate how people's choices tend to be mixed for normal illness and tend to focus on remedies based within the private sphere. For instance, in Donovan's (1986) study of Afro-Caribbean and South Asian women in East London, women in the study used remedies such as herbal teas: Herbs were boiled and taken for coughs and colds and asthma. This is also supported by Helman's (1978) classic study of the archetypal British complaint, the common cold, which was focused on a whole complex of beliefs including ideas related to food, such as "feed a cold, starve a fever." Within my study, women's views about general illness tended to be by and large syncretic, with a heavier weighting toward the use of non-Western remedies. This can be seen to be "private" syncrecy; that is, syncrecy located mostly within the domestic realm and drawing on remedies that are food related but also related to Asian medical systems.

When I asked my respondents how they dealt with general illness such as colds they referred almost explicitly to their use of home remedies. These remedies included remedies that were not specifically from Asian medicine, and quite often related to various teas, garlic capsules, or herbs from the garden. As Charlotte, an Indo-Caribbean Catholic, pointed out:

> I make ginger tea. I swear by that, it's usually really good for treating colds and things.

As the following quote from Sakeena shows, while the remedies respondents used for colds were not always specifically associated with Asian medical systems, they were related by the women to their cultural and religious background, particularly to diet:

> If it's a cough, a little bit of Turmeric powder in milk before we go to bed and drink that. I do that regularly. Honey is also very good and it's in our religious book [Koran] as well that there's a cure in honey, if we have bruises.

The health choices of respondents surrounding colds and coughs were particularly syncretic, as they also used remedies for colds associated with Western health care. Kishwar, a Muslim, like many of the women also discussed the crossovers between remedies. She suggested that Western and non-Western health care could not be seen as completely separate:

> I mean, with coughs we'd use lemsip. That helps a lot and also for sore throats, honey and lemon and stuff which I make myself with herbs and remedies from the kitchen.

This syncretic use of remedies is again reflected in other studies on lay attitudes to health. In Helman's (1978) study, while using herbal and home remedies for fevers, people often used antibiotics at the same time. Similarly, in Donovan's (1986) study the respondents often mixed remedies; for example, using a mix of almond powders and milk and apple jam, anadin for headaches, panadol and lemon tea for flu. As Helman (1978) argues, there is an interaction between biomedicine and folk ideas on general illness. From this it appears that most lay populations draw on a plurality of remedies for general illnesses. Within my study, however, the women's position as British Asians gave them access to a particular set of non-Western Asian remedies not open to the general population of Britain. As women socialized within British culture, they also had greater knowledge and access to resources within Western medicine that more recently migrated women (such as those in Donovan's study) are excluded from.

Under the guise of general health, respondents also talked about illnesses such as stomach bugs, general nausea, and diarrhea and outlined the remedies they often used for such ills. Surinder, a Sikh, discussed the use of a whole plethora of herbs and food-related remedies for such illnesses:

> If you have a mild tummy ache then use fennel, you take water with it. If you've got an ear infection as well just put some garlic and some mustard oil, then just heat that up and put a drop of that in the ear and it clears it up.

What was interesting within the accounts of the women studied was their significant use of Asian balms for a whole number of general illnesses. The women's location in Leicester can be seen to influence such use of balms like "tiger balm" for general illnesses. As will be shown in Chapter 5, many Asian health products were available in Leicester. Women felt that this related to the city's multiculturalism and large Asian population. They felt that they could access Indian and other Asian health goods in Leicester that were less available in other parts of Britain.

Such balms can be used for a wide range of illness, from colds to rheumatism. Shahnaz and Samina, both Muslim, point out their wide-ranging usage:

Tiger balm, you can use it for rheumatic pains or whatever you know, muscular pains, especially good for colds and flus and you know, you get sweaty, sweat your germs out.

I use that on my back a lot. It doesn't cure it really but it gives you that comfort at the time. It's really hot stuff, very strong.

Sharma (1992) identifies pain and in particular back pain (along with allergies) as the most frequent problems for which people seek alternative care. Regarding aches and pains associated with general illnesses, while favoring non-Western remedies the women's accounts emphasized a use of syncretic remedies, both Western and non-Western, within the domestic realm. Women within the study also used their non-Western remedies with general remedies, often bought from the pharmacist. For instance, Rhamba's husband had back problems. He used a combination of Asian balms and an anti-inflammatory drug:

My husband he has back pain, a back tumour or abscess whatever it is. He finds Ibuprofen makes it feel better so I keep Ibuprofen, Co-Codamol and Paracetamol.

Women within the study also used a plurality of medicines for conditions that were recurring but did not necessarily require day-to-day management. This often took the women out of the domestic realm to seek out public Asian medical practitioners. This emphasizes a shift from the domestic to the public domain as illness becomes slightly more concerning. For instance, Kishwar discussed her husband's use of Chinese medicine for hayfever:

I have taken my husband to a Chinese herbalist on Evington Road. That's to do with his hayfever. He suffers so badly with his hayfever, so we've tried that.

As the second account from Kishwar shows, however, this was used in conjunction with Western remedies within the home, emphasizing the women's use of syncretic medicines for general health issues:

> His Western medicine helps but he has to take so many tablets so he decided to go to a healer as well.

In terms of health choices, the women in the study talked mostly about ill health and health problems rather than about health itself. In the absence of illness women talked a little about remedies they used in order to maintain health. Healthy lifestyles are promulgated by the medical profession and health promoters (Blaxter 1990). The links made between lifestyles and health reflect broader social changes and are linked to the rise of consumer culture (Nettleton 1995). In this respect there is a commercialization of health in that people are constructed as health consumers who may consume healthy lifestyles. At the center of this is body maintenance (for example, exercise and food) (Featherstone 1991; Nettleton 1995).[2] Within this study, women mostly talked about maintaining good health through diet, as Shahnaz shows:

> Yes, I do tend to control it [diet] because a lot of it [ill health] we believe is through your diet. You know, we do try because there are a lot of unhealthy foods as well that are available in Indian cooking, but as I say it's down to you basically.

Hindu women in the study, such as Musarat, were mostly vegetarian and associated such a diet with good health. Many of the women within the study had syncretic diets, eating a mix of both Western and non-Western foods:

> Yes, I cook mostly Indian foods yes, once or twice I'll make lasagne or something like that. We're mixed, I make Indian foods but I also make pasta and things like that.

Some of the respondents, such as Sakeena, used home remedies on a daily basis in order to prevent ill health:

Yeah, and what I believe is each month, three days in a row every morning if you have honey you won't suffer from any serious illness.

On the whole, for general illness few women within the study consulted either their general practitioner (GP) or Hakims or Vaidas.[3] As Miles (1991) argues, the common response to conditions that are familiar and seem minor, such as coughs, colds, and headaches, is to ignore the problem in the hope that it will go away and prove temporary and insignificant. Worsley (1997) points out that for minor illnesses even today, people consult their GPs only about one in five times they feel ill. For common symptoms, including high temperature, arthritis, anemia, and sore throat, people consult pharmacists, self-help groups, and health cults. Advice seeking goes beyond consulting any kind of professional. The women in this study were likely to consult a doctor about general illness only if symptoms continued after the women had attempted to treat themselves at home.

The women's use of various types of medicine for different types of illness was also temporally located. For example, the respondents' choices around colds and flu were fluid and not fixed. Rambha's account shows how initially people treat general illness at home, but when it does not clear up they may resort to the doctor.

What I do for the first couple of days is get something over the counter or mixtures or something like that before I go to the doctor.

Initially the women might make certain choices for a particular illness, but these may change as time passes. As women become more familiar with particular types of illness, they may stop using Western treatments and start using Asian home remedies or healers instead. As will be shown in Chapter 3, this intersects with the change in women's social circumstances. As women progress throughout the life course, get married, become mothers, and so on their health choices change. Inder discusses her change in attitude toward illness in relation to her children having colds:

> Initially I took her [her daughter] straight around to the doctor's a lot, for colds and stuff. I just stop taking her and now I make them [her children] stuff at home, hot lemon and honey, milk and things like that.

Again, the women in the study suggested that this reflected a broader trend within society where people were increasingly looking for quick-fix solutions to general illness. From the women's accounts it became important to recognize that while their choices might be syncretic for particular illnesses this cannot be fixed in time, as choices change over time and as women pass through the life course. This was particularly true relating to normal illness and seemed to be because women suffered general ills frequently and so became more used to dealing with them. The women were less likely to talk about temporal shifts in health choices in the same way relating to real illness. Other research has shown that age and experience is a key factor in shifting responses to chronic illness over time (Bury and Holme 1991). By the time people have survived into their seventies and eighties, experience may have equipped them to deal with and adapt to new situations such as chronic illness (Pound, Gompertz, and Ebrahim 1998; Williams 2000). This relates to position within the life course; the older a person is, the more that person becomes used to certain types of illness. For the women within this study, real illnesses were things to be feared. While women's attitudes over more manageable types of real illness (e.g., diabetes) might change as the illnesses become part of life, for fatal illness health choices, while not fixed in time, seemed to be far less open to change. This, however, reflected the respondents' position within the life course and may well change as women grow older.

HEALTH PROBLEMS:
BETWEEN HEALTH AND ILLNESS

Cornwell (1984), within her tripartite categorization system, talks about health problems. Health problems are not necessarily illnesses; they are problems associated with natural processes of aging and the reproductive cycle and problems that are thought to stem from a person's nature or personality, such as allergies, asthma, and eczema. She argues that the common feature of this category of problems is that they are thought not to be amenable to medical treatment. Sometimes some forms of self-treatment may be advocated. There are those associated with growing old (e.g., varicose veins) and those associated with menstruation, pregnancy, and menopause (e.g., abdominal pain, depression, and dizziness). As mentioned earlier, the category of health problems is particularly relevant to women. One must apply caution here in locating these health problems as women's problems. There has been a long history of linking madness with so-called feminine traits and relating the condition to women's reproductive roles (Showalter 1987). This filters through in much contemporary health literature to equations of women's health with reproductive health (see Chapter 3), and to contestation surrounding women's overrepresentation within statistics on mental health (Pilgrim and Rogers 1993).[4]

Women within the study talked frequently about health issues such as pregnancy and depression and anxiety. They seemed to see these as transgressing the health–illness binary, as not quite being one thing or the other, as being somehow "improper" illnesses. This applies to issues relating to mental illness in the sense that these belong within the psychological not the physical realm, physical illness constituting "real" illness. It applies to the women's views on reproduction and gynecological issues because these were seen in many senses as natural processes and part of women's lot. Respondents' health choices surrounding these health issues were complex and diverse, depending on the particular type of health problem. Within the women's accounts it seemed that as an interstitial category health issues felt to be health problems had the potential to fluctuate between the category of health problems, a state of natural health, through normal illness, to real illness. Because of such fluctuations the respondents' health choices ranged freely within this category. In most ways they were syncretic, drawing on Western and non-Western remedies. This syncrecy was relational to time and context, highlighting the importance of both in influencing health choices.

Anxiety, Depression, and Spirituality

It has been a consistent finding of researchers and confirmed by health practitioners that lay people have uncertain and often ambivalent and contradictory views about the meaning of mental disturbance and whether to regard it as an illness or not (Miles 1991). When talking about illness, Cornwell's (1984) respondents meant physical illness. When they talked about anxiety and depression they meant these as states of mind consigned to the category of health problems. Other studies have also demonstrated a split in ideas between mental and physical illness (Donovan 1986), and discussed varying definitions of what constitutes anxiety and depression cross-culturally (Fenton and Sadiq-Sangster 1996).

Several women within this study talked about feeling depressed or anxious at particular points and sought out various non-Western and Western medical and religious remedies as a response. Within the study, however, women did not talk in terms of "mental health" generally, but instead spoke about mental health issues, using terms such as depression and anxiety. They saw depression as fairly common and nothing to be ashamed or fearful of. Depression appeared to be defined by the women as a health problem. When talking about mental health issues, women in the study seemed to make a mind–body split. Mental health was seen as something quite separate from physical health. Women made this split and then based their use of particular remedies accordingly.

Shahnaz makes the distinction between the ways in which physical and mental illness are both perceived and treated:

> Some things aren't sorted by the GP. When you've got something straightforward, physical, you know, when you've got a broken arm or leg or something the doctor can help. But sometimes, with other mental problems they just try and keep you drowsy, you know, docile, they're not actually facing the problem.

Again, the women's views were syncretic but tended to be biased toward non-Western medicine. This use of different remedies was also related mostly to the public realm. In cases of mental health problems respondents' quite often went to non-Western or religious healers. Such healers seemed to be readily available to the women in Leicester. While they might also go to the doctor for antidepressants, their faith lay mostly with religious healers, taking a "prayer and Prozac" approach (Matthews and Larson 1997).[5] This was particularly true for Muslim women. As Shahnaz shows in relation to her mother's depression,

> My mother suffers from depression and she's seeing a religious person for that. But it's had some effects. She's on medication as well from the doctor but she's also seeing a religious person.

Other research on mental health has shown that it is common for women to turn to religion and religious healers in times of emotional distress (Donovan 1986). Hillier and Rahman (1996) studied Bangladeshi perceptions of childhood behavioral and emotional problems in Tower Hamlets, London. They found that at times of mental illness, while doctors were the most favored ports of call in both the United Kingdom and Bangladesh, this was followed very closely by the mullah (religious healer) and persons at the mosque. They concluded that while in general people are open minded about Western medicine, they are not uncritical. They accept it works for some kinds of physical illness and for other common and serious conditions (e.g., arthritis, neuralgia), but it is less effective when dealing with psychosomatic problems ranging from heartbreak to witchcraft.

Within my study there appeared a multilayering of types of problems associated with anxiety and depression and other emotional problems. Many of these were often related to being possessed by spirits, although possession by spirits could cause other "physically" located health problems as well. As Samina's account shows, when women suspected possession by spirits, religious healers were often sought:

Spiritual healers they usually deal with things that are spiritually wrong with you. You know if there is something like depression that's really common now and some people think, well she's probably possessed or something, or there's something wrong with her or the house she lives in whatever.

While the women often sought public figures in the form of religious healers in dealing with these types of mental health problems, they also carried out particular religious practices at home in order to rid the afflicted person of their possession. These practices within the private realm were related to practices associated with the evil eye (see Chapters 3 and 4). For Gurinder, a Sikh respondent, spiritual remedies were something to be cautious of:

I wouldn't try it because some of the remedies are really superstitious like the evil eye.

Researchers have often linked such lay use of non-Western (particularly spiritual) medicine for mental health problems with the inadequacies of biomedicine. Fernando (1991) ties this to the psychiatric profession having little or no interest in cultural issues. He attributes this to the mechanistic model that dominates Western psychiatry. Biomedicine is seen to have no place for illness brought on by supernatural forces (Worsley 1997). In talking about Asian migrants in the United States, Loue (1999) highlights a reluctance for people to utilize the health services for mental health issues. These are often deemed inappropriate and preferred techniques are often found in prayer or various traditional remedies. Worsley (1997) also supports this argument, suggesting that the insensitivity of biomedicine often leads people to turn to other forms of hope and comfort—diviners, shamans, and religious specialists—for disorders that are believed to arise when people's social relations are out of kilter. Non-Western medical systems theorize about mental illness in a completely different manner than biomedicine. Ayurvedic medicines and Unani distinguish between mental illness caused by sorcery, that caused by evil spirits or ghosts, and a disease described as "malfunctioning of the head," often produced by shocks or setbacks in life (Bhattacharya 1986; Hillier and Rahman 1996). As already suggested, women's accounts emphasize this multilayering of causes of problems such as depression. Women within the study talked about the inadequacies of biomedicine in dealing with mental health problems, but not quite as strictly as the model presented here suggests. It seemed in many women's cases it had more to do with following their faith and a drawing on the health choices of previous generations.

There was a split within the women's accounts between those who used religion and religious healers for depression and those that did not. This split was made along religious lines. It was mostly Muslim women within the research who sought out spiritual healers for mental health, although Sikh women talked about them to some extent. The Hindu women within the project seemed on the whole to talk about depression less. Also, while two Hindu women had either suffered mental health problems themselves or had family members who had, they had sought out Western health remedies and care and focused on keeping themselves busy. As Ramila, a Hindu respondent, points out,

I never used to go before (to the doctors) but now I go all
the time because I'm suffering from depression. I go
every six weeks for a check up, talk about how I'm feeling, get checked out.

Later in the interview I asked Ramila how she dealt with her
depression:

I just keep myself busy. If I stayed at home all the time.
I'd keep going over things in my mind, keep on crying
and things like that. I just stay busy and take him [her
son] out.

Religious difference among respondents relating to their
health choices highlights the heterogeneity of the category
"South Asian." Religious difference is one example of such
heterogeneity. Such religious difference in health choice is
something that will be explored further in Chapter 4. Regarding depression and other related issues, it was not just a
case of the women drawing on either Western biomedicine
or non-Western health remedies. While the women would
use doctors and Western medicines for depression, they
seemed eager to find other ways of dealing with it. This also
ties in with the amorphous nature of mental health problems like anxiety and depression and their position as "health
problems" and not "real" illness; similar comparisons can
be made in this sense with pregnancy.

Several of the women specifically located the cause of their
depression within their social circumstances. For instance,
some women within the study did display signs of depression relating particularly to feelings of isolation brought about
by being at home alone. Just under half of the women within
the study were housewives at home with small children.
Several other women worked in part-time employment and
suffered from feelings of isolation bought on by long periods
spent at home. This relates to the argument made by Brown
and Harris (1978) relating women's positions and roles within
society to a higher incidence of depression. In this sense, the

lay referral network regarding depression was an invaluable tool for respondents. The lay referral network is a network that provides health solutions and information about when and how to seek medical advice. It is made up of husbands, relatives, and friends. Talking about their problems with those closest to them was a useful way for the women to deal with their health problems. Previous research has also suggested the importance of the lay referral network in influencing women's treatment of mental health problems such as depression. Women suffering from depression frequently report having talked to other women about feeling low, not coping, or sleeplessness before going to the doctor (Miles 1991).

Overall, the women's accounts of mental health issues such as depression can be seen to be syncretic. Women within the study used both Western and non-Western remedies when dealing with issues such as depression. Women's use of these remedies was also not restricted specifically to either the private or public domains, but incorporated both. While choices were syncretic, though, there was higher weighting toward their use of non-Western remedies. If we move on to look at other types of health problems, such as pregnancy and other gynecological issues, women can also be seen to use syncretic remedies with a heavy weighting to non-Western medicine. By looking at these other problems we can also highlight the complexity and fluidity of the category of health problems and see the effects of this on health choices.

Contradictions and Conflicts: Menstruation and Pregnancy

Gynecological and reproductive health issues also fall under the guise of "health problems." Concurring with Cornwell (1984) and other studies (Graham and Oakley 1986; Scambler and Scambler 1993), women in my study tended to identify period pains and pregnancy as somewhere in-between health and ill health. Again, these types of health problems can be seen to occupy interstitial spaces. Pregnancy in particular can be seen to shift in and out of different categories of illness.

Menstruation, like pregnancy, is surrounded by ambiguities and uncertainties. Although it is a normal healthy function of the female body, it causes pain and discomfort. Menstruation is described as "the blossoming of the red flower" in many vernacular traditions, and referred to as "period" or "monthly" by doctors or health workers and as "being down" by many adolescents (Chhachhi and Price 1998, 102). Periods are both pathologized within medical literature and seen as part of normal life (Martin 1989). According to Scambler and Scambler (1985) in a British study, women's perceptions of menstruation have to be considered in the context of deeply rooted social and cultural beliefs. They note that perceptions surrounding menstruation differ widely in different societies. In the accounts of the women studied here, there seemed to be a certain coyness around the whole issue. Women seemed to feel that they really needed to just "get on with it" rather than make a fuss about pain and tension associated with menstruation. These notions of getting on with it fit in with the findings of other studies on women and menstruation (Blaxter 1983). Respondents felt that period pains should not be seen as a problem. It was just a case of keeping comfortable. As Surinder points out,

> I mean for period pains, it's just a hot water bottle which is as much for comfort as it is for pain, so just that.

None of the women researched consulted the doctor about their periods, and anything used to comfort women during this time was either bought from the pharmacist or taken from the kitchen cupboard.

Miles (1991) argues that women's views on pregnancy tend to be characterized by ambiguity. Is it health or illness? Pregnancy and childbirth are often presented as both (Woollett and Marshall 1997). As a consequence, women struggle to attach meaning to their experiences and to ascertain the socially approved and appropriate ways to behave. Women receive conflicting messages from doctors and other health professionals, from their relations and friends, and from their own bodies. During their early teen years girls often assimilate the view of pregnancy as a natural state, part of womanhood and femininity. This is then often contradicted by the message from health professionals that pregnancy is a medical state that needs to be checked and monitored by doctors and obstetricians in hospital prenatal clinics, all of whom treat pregnant women as if ill. Uncertainties about the nature of pregnancy are also aroused by the bodily sensations of pain and discomfort that many women experience (Graham and Oakley 1986).

During pregnancy this interstitial positioning between health and ill health often leads women to draw on lay advice from friends and relatives. Many changes in lifestyle are advocated and tried: taking certain types of exercise, eating in specific ways, resting more or less. Such measures are often attractive because they can be tried without seeking expert advice (Miles 1991). Regarding pregnancy, studies have demonstrated a revival of interest among women in traditional remedies in the United Kingdom and the United States (Chamberlain 1981). Minor illnesses and discomforts during the natural biological process are treated by many women in this way. Homans (1985) found that in her sample the majority of British Asian women (73%, mostly Punjabi) used traditional remedies for the discomforts of pregnancy, which they usually learned from older female relatives. White women in the same study were less likely to have the relevant information, but even among them 35 percent knew and used folk remedies (milk, lemonade, polo, roughage in the diet, almond, ginger, and many other remedies for stomach problems in pregnancy).

The women's views on pregnancy within my study were very eclectic, involving syncretic health choices. For pregnancy, though, it was not simply that women used both Western and non-Western health remedies. It also related to the status of pregnancy as both health and illness, as occupying a space between the two, moving in and out of both categories. This led women in the study to draw on a whole plethora of medicines; not just those related to health systems and remedies, but also those that are socially and culturally embedded, relating particularly to diet and located in religious beliefs. As with the findings of other studies (Homans 1985; Woollett and Dosanjh-Matwala 1990), food was particularly important within the research. Women within the study explained their food choices not just in terms of nausea and sickness, but also in terms of hot and cold in the Ayurvedic–Unani tibb systems of medicine and in their cultural context. Shahnaz demonstrates when talking about food choice:

> Hot and cold, but not actually physically hot and physically cold but the way it reacts to you like certain things like, like milk is supposed to help you cool down isn't it? Bananas are meant to help you cool down but there are other types of food that are supposed to make you sweat [aubergines], "hot" but not hot in temperature, or in spiciness or anything like that.

Many of the women within the study ate different "hot" and "cold" foods at different stages of the pregnancy. Older women (mothers) encouraged women trying to conceive to eat cool foods:

> When you are trying to conceive a baby, trying to get pregnant they tell us to stop eating warm things like carrots and aubergines, ginger etc. they tell us rather just to have lots of milkshakes. They say the womb needs to be at a cool temperature to conceive.

The women were actively encouraged not to eat hot foods at this time and early into pregnancy, as this might lead to miscarriage. This stood in opposition to later stages of pregnancy, where respondents were encouraged to eat hot foods to ease labor. This occurred from about six or seven months on, as Sakeena explains:

When you're nine months, you should start eating foods which are hot and slippery. Slippery means like if you put a little bit of ghee or butter in your meal, so it helps the baby come quickly.

Similarly, the women were encouraged to eat certain (hot) foods after the birth to encourage bleeding, which signifies a clearing out of the system. Samina discusses what foods you are supposed to eat postnatally:

After we have given birth they [mother or elders] make us this drink which has fennel seeds in it and they put this special brown sugar stuff in it, you put it in water with a bit of ghee. They make us this to help us clear out our system because we want a period after we've had our babies so that makes it all come out. It tastes horrible but it really helps to clear out your system.

The influence of hot and cold foods was also applied by Muslim women within the study to other gynecological problems. Samina discusses the use of hot and cold foods for cystitis:

Yes, if a woman suffers from cystitis and that, that's when they tell you to have cold things like yogurt and milk and milkshakes.

Within Donovan's (1986) study, South Asian respondents talked about the relationship between hot and cold foods and certain illnesses, although not particularly pregnancy. This was more in terms of keeping a healthy balance. A normal temperature signals health. Any deviation from this is seen to indicate some sort of ill health. Some illnesses and diseases were defined by Donovan's informants to be hot and cold and balance was restored in the body by taking hot and cold foods to cancel out excess. For instance, if you have a high temperature use a cold compound to bring temperature down; measles is a hot disease so you cannot eat hot foods like meat, eggs, chicken, and so on. Within my study, women's discussions of hot and cold foods was more or less tied to issues of pregnancy and reproductive health and did not really feature in women's accounts regarding other health issues.

While Hindu and Sikh women within the study did not eat foods that had hot or cold properties during pregnancy, they did try to eat particular foods. Sita discusses the various foods you are supposed to eat when pregnant to keep healthy:

> When you're pregnant, you're supposed to have lots of milk, nuts and cheese. They're supposed to be really good for you.

All the women within the study continued to use a variety of remedies used for normal illness for the various associated symptoms of pregnancy, such as balms and the like. All the women's accounts demonstrated the importance of the lay referral network on health choices. This emphasizes the way in which the influence of illness cannot be divorced from people's social and cultural contexts. Rather, the women's accounts highlight the socially and culturally embedded nature of illness itself. Other studies have also highlighted the significance of women's wider social relations during pregnancy, such as friends and work colleagues (Woollett and Marshall 1997).Women within the study also talked about the influence of their social networks on their health choices during pregnancy. However, they did not discuss the role of their husbands and partners in the context of pregnancy. This is at odds with other studies on women and pregnancy, which have highlighted the significance of men's roles (Woollett and Marshall 1997). Within this study, women talked mostly about the significant influence of their mothers and older female relations on their use of various remedies during pregnancy. Sakeena says,

> But you know, if you are living with an older person they will stop you from doing this or that, most of the ladies tend to listen because older women have experience.

Rambha's account also demonstrates her mother's influence regarding advice for general symptoms. She talks about this in relation to indigestion during pregnancy:

> I used to say to my mum, "should I take anything?" and my mum used to say, "no don't take anything, just have a glass of juice and lie down that's it and have small not big meals."

While generational influence on health choices will be explored in more detail in Chapter 3, it is worth noting here that the women in this study usually took their own mothers' advice on issues relating to pregnancy.

All the women within the study had regular checkups with a general practitioner during pregnancy and had their children in the hospital. The women's accounts suggested, though, that pregnancy was not something to keep bothering the doctor over, that it was part of a woman's lot. Homans (1985) noted that Asian women (from the Punjab, Gujarat) living in Britain were less likely than White women to go to the doctor with complaints during pregnancy, but she argued that this may be changing as other sources of help decline (family ties breaking down). The difficulties experienced by Black and Hispanic women seeking help from White doctors in Britain and the United States may well result in their becoming reluctant seekers of help (Miles 1991). Many studies have highlighted the various ways in which Black women experience racism during prenatal care (Bowler 1993; Bowes and Domokos 1996). For instance, Bowler (1993) highlights the stereotyping of South Asian women by hospital midwives. Bowes and Domokos's (1996) research among Pakistani women in Glasgow also highlights the wide-ranging experiences of racism by individual women in their study. Women often felt they were being viewed in a stereotypical manner. One of their respondents who usually wore Western clothes explained why she wore *shalwar chameez* (Punjabi dress) to the antenatal clinic: "I will wear these clothes, and open my mouth later on to shock people you know, shock

white people, because they think this is an idiot sitting there
wearing these clothes" (p. 58).

From the accounts of the women within the study, it seems
clear that cultural norms, past experiences with doctors, and
the existence of alternative help sources were more influential factors on seeking medical help than the doctor's actual
ability to deal with the symptoms. This could in some ways
explain why the women's use of non-Western remedies during pregnancy is restricted to the domestic realm. However,
women within this study were reluctant to talk about racism
as an issue for not visiting the doctor. This may concur with
Bowes and Domokos's (1996) study, where negative experiences by women were not always perceived as being due to
racism.

Within the study women seemed to suggest their use of
non-Western remedies within the domestic realm was different to anything suggested through the care they received
within Western medicine. Shahnaz said, on the use of hot
and cold foods,

> There are certain types of foods and things that you are
> supposed to have after birth to help clear out the body.
> We believe, and I don't know if this is Western thought
> as well but I've never heard a midwife tell you this, but
> the more you bleed, the better it is for you because you
> get rid of everything. All of that build up inside you.

The women seemed to state these differences but did not
seem to see them necessarily as an imposition of biomedical
views onto the women during the prenatal phase, as suggested by Karseras and Hopkins (1987). Respondents never
presented these differences as outright conflict between types
of medicine, although there seemed to be potential for this.
It was more the case that both private and public and Western and non-Western medicine were held in conjunction.

Charlotte was the only woman within the study to talk
about postnatal depression. The doctor put her on antidepressants:

I'm a lot calmer person now. I went through horrendous postnatal depression with my first and then after the caesarean I was really upset because I hadn't come to terms with it. I went to the doctors and he put me on medication and I couldn't believe it I was like, three months down the line and I could see a tunnel. I could see things clearly for the first time in my life. I'm actually more focused now than I've ever been.

Pregnancy was experienced by most of the women as a natural state or health problem. Pregnancy can also at times creep into the category of normal illness, as women have symptoms that fit into this category (e.g., indigestion). For most of the respondents pregnancy rarely went into the category of real illness; however, for a few women pregnancy became classified as a serious illness that required long-term periods of hospitalization, as Deepika's account shows:

During the pregnancy I was really ill. The last few months I had to stay in hospital. It was really frightening for a while both mine and my baby's health was really compromised.

When pregnancy moved into the realm of serious illness, respondents' health choices ceased being syncretic and moved completely into the realm of Western health care (this is something picked up later in the context of "real" illness).

Within this section, the women's accounts can be seen to highlight the significant intersection of illness with social context. The women's choices regarding pregnancy are often couched within their social relations, particularly drawing on their relationships with their mothers. The women use a range of remedies for pregnancy, access to which must also be related to their broader position as British Asians. As Asian women who are part of a globally dispersed ethnic group, respondents have greater access to certain non-Western remedies. As British born they can be seen to have greater bargaining power within biomedicine than those who have migrated more recently to Britain from India and elsewhere. Through the women's accounts, health problems can be seen to occupy interstitial spaces, moving between different types of medicine, both Western and non-Western and private and public.

MANAGING ILLNESS:
SHIFTS TO WESTERN MEDICINE

Cornwell's (1984) third category of illness is termed "real" illness. The model for real illness is established by the major and "modern" disabling and life-threatening diseases (i.e., cancers and cardiovascular and coronary heart diseases). The reality of the illness is established by the poor prognosis and by the impact it makes on the patient. Epilepsy, diabetes, and other chronic disabling diseases, which require constant medication, are included. Real illness definitely falls within the province of medicine, but that is not to say that all illness in this category is treatable (Miles 1991). The definition refers to the severity and therefore the status of the condition rather than to whether or not medical treatment actually exists or is successful.

A similar categorization of serious illness is made within this study along the lines of Cornwell's (1984) category of real illness. In opposition to health choices for normal illness, women drew almost exclusively on Western medicine for serious illness. Such choices are common among lay persons, even for those with wide access to non-Western medicine. As Guo (2000) argues in his study on aging Chinese people in Flushing, New York, while people might use traditional Chinese medicine for a variety of ills, anything listed by his respondents as "big problems" were taken care of by biomedical doctors. Within this section of the chapter I have focused on three types of manageable and serious illnesses prevalent within the women's accounts: asthma, diabetes, and cancers and fatal illness.

Particularly strong links have been made regarding the benefits of "alternative" medicine for diseases such as diabetes and asthma (British Holistic Medical Association 1992). Within this study, for illnesses that required daily management, such as asthma and eczema, women drew much more heavily on Western medicine. Although at times they might use Asian medicine, there was an ultimate deferral to Western medicine. This went for illnesses such as asthma, eczema, and diabetes. Asthma was identified by many of the women as a key problem associated with living in Leicester, a city with pollution problems. It seemed mostly to be prevalent among the women's children.

The women did try to control these types of illnesses at home to a certain extent because most of them were not happy about children's long-term use of steroids, either in treatment for eczema or in inhalers for asthma. Respondents often related this "home treatment" to having particular types of diet to reduce the prevalence of asthma attacks. Donovan's (1986) study also suggests this. Her respondents drew on ideas about hot and cold foods that were supposed to be used in the treatment of asthma. Too many cold foods and drinks could have very serious side effects for asthmatics. Many of her respondents felt that cold things like ice cream and cold drinks in winter led to illnesses such as pneumonia. Inder's account within my study about her daughter's asthma supports this. She was quite keen to control the asthma through diet rather than have her daughter dependent on an inhaler:

> My eldest daughter seems to be getting a touch of asthma and eczema. The doctor recommends an inhaler but I've said no. . . . I've found that when she's having problems with her breathing, drinking tea and things helps, so she just has tea and coffee and other warm drinks rather than coke.

Some women in the study did use non-Western practitioners such as Hakims for things like eczema and asthma, although respondents often complained that these treatments were too expensive. Regarding such illnesses, a conflict in treatments often develops between Western and non-Western remedies, leading to a focus on Western medicine. This will be explored in more detail in the next chapter.

Diabetes has long been seen as a disease of immigrant populations and in particular South Asian populations. Pitchumon and Saran (1976) identified a high rate of diabetes among South Asians within the United States as well as in Asians located in East Africa. Within the United Kingdom studies have also focused on the high incidence of diabetes among the South Asian population (Kelleher and Islam 1996). Explanations for such rates have ranged from the suggestion of some type of genetic disposition to the disease to an association with the effects brought about by a lifestyle change through migration. There have also been a number of studies that explored minority use of different types of medicine for the management of diabetes. Armstrong and Pierce (1996) argue in their study on diabetes among Afro-Caribbean populations in Brixton that there was no mention of folk remedies. The converse is found to be true in other studies on Afro-Caribbean health choice (Donovan 1986). Regarding studies on diabetes among Asian populations in Britain, Kelleher and Islam (1996), in their study of Bangladeshis in Tower Hamlets, found a minimal use of non-Western medicine.

Women within this study held attitudes about diabetes that were similar to those held about asthma. If anything, they were even more reluctant to use non-Western products in order to try and control it. Many women had some family member who was diabetic and felt that they would only really trust a general practitioner and Western medicine. Only one woman, Gurinder, knew of someone who had tried Asian medical products for diabetes, and this was during a trip to India and did not help at all:

> My mum, she has diabetes and she tried herbal tablets in India. The treatment for diabetes is free and you have to take it for forty days and apparently you're supposed to cut out on a lot of things. You have it for forty days and you're supposed to get rid of diabetes and my mum didn't do it properly and didn't get rid of hers.

Other studies on the incidence of diabetes among Asian populations in Britain have pointed to the control of diet and particularly the use of karella, a bitter vegetable, in the management of diabetes. Kelleher and Islam (1996) found that karella was widely used. In their study some of the respondents said that they had been told by doctors to use karella and claimed that it was on the hospital diet sheet, which is an example of doctors being able to work with lay ideas. There is some evidence that karella does help to lower blood sugar levels, which helped to persuade doctors to accept it (Kelleher and Islam 1996). Diet control, though, was in all cases used in conjunction with insulin dependence.

Women within the study were aware of karella. Some women did at times try and "help" diabetes through diet, and some talked about the use of karella to help lower sugar levels. Samina discusses the uses of karella:

> There's this long vegetable, like long cucumbers with horrible skin [karella]. They're really horrible and bitter the juices out of that; they [diabetics] have the juices out of that. To prevent, well to make sugar levels low. Having a teaspoon of that every morning before your breakfast because my dad has diabetes and he uses that.

Within the women's accounts of diabetes, however, there did not seem to be a significant interconnection between GPs and the home use of karella. On the whole, the respondents in Kelleher and Islam's (1996) study saw their diabetes as a problem that had to be managed medically. They did not appear to think that forest or folk remedies had much to offer them, apart from the widely used karella. Within this study, Rambha's view of preferring to draw almost completely on Western medicine for the treatment of diabetes was quite common among the women:

> He [her brother-in-law] was quite recently diagnosed [with diabetes] then the daughter. They knew what it was as soon as they got the symptoms, starting to go to

the loo and stuff a lot. Yeah, she's going to the doctor's all the time because she's insulin dependent. She has to be careful what she eats, you feel sorry for her but yeah; it has to be treated by the doctors.

The extended family in Rambha's case were sensitive to the needs of diabetes sufferers. As the aunt of a diabetic child, Rambha kept diabetic foods in the house for when her niece was visiting.

Regarding children's health, studies have shown a high incidence of use of alternative medicine for serious illnesses such as cancer (Bridgen 1995). Respondents in my study were reluctant to speak about serious illnesses such as cancer and appeared surprised when I asked whether they would consider using non-Western health care. Respondents would talk in a roundabout way about cancer within the family, but always in terms of Western care. Women within the study seemed to have ultimate faith in Western medicine. This concurs with some of the attitudes of respondents in Donovan's (1986) study; all her respondents were afraid of getting a serious illness such as a stroke, cancer, or losing a limb. Many of the informants cited cancer as an incurable disease, but revealed great faith in Western medicine and doctors. Acceptance of what happens and faith in Western medicine comes through in some women's statements.

With regard to serious illness such as cancer, the women here went directly to Western health care. Non-Western health care would be sought out only occasionally, if Western medicine proved ineffective over a certain period of time. This can be seen in an account from Shahnaz about her brother-in-law. He had been very ill with his stomach and had failed to be properly diagnosed in the United Kingdom so went to India to be diagnosed and have treatment (using Western health care there, though). In India he was diagnosed immediately with stomach cancer and given chemotherapy, but unfortunately the treatment failed to save him:

He got the tumors removed in India. He was prescribed a dose of chemotherapy there. He came home to Leicester and they wouldn't give him the dose prescribed in India. Within three months his symptoms were back.

This man also did use some "alternatives" in India relating to Asian medical systems, but this seemed like it might be a last-ditch attempt in the face of such unsatisfactory treatment and was not wholly relied upon. In studies focusing on the use of alternative medicine for cancer, reasons for using alternative medicines have fallen into two main categories: (1) patients are "pushed" toward alternatives because of bad experiences with conventional medical treatment, or (2) patients are "pulled" toward alternative medicine because of their belief in the alternative paradigm (Furnham and Smith 1988).Within this study, reasons for using non-Western medicine definitely fell within the first category and it appeared that using non-Western medicine was a last resort. To go back to the example of Shahnaz,

> I mean you can see with my brother-in-law, he did actually get some medications from India, religious. But I think you do tend to use them but you can't rely on them.

As will be shown in Chapter 5, women felt that their position as British Asian women gave them access to medical systems in other contexts. This at least offered them more health options than those presented to many White English people, even if, as in the case of Shahnaz, treatment proves ineffective. This highlights the ways in which illness intersects with ethnicity to influence health choices, and again emphasizes the ways in which health choices must be situated within the social context of people's lives.

CONCLUSION

This discussion has been centered around the conceptualization of health and illness, exploring the ways in which such conceptualization affects health choices. As Cornwell (1984) argues, it is common for people to categorize illness.

In her research and also within this study illness can roughly be divided into three categories: normal illness, health problems, and real illness. Within the context of this research, such categorization has in turn influenced women's use of Western and non-Western medicines. The women drew syncretically on a range of medicines for normal illness and health problems; for real illness, however, they were more likely to draw solely on Western medicine.

In focusing on the conceptualization of health and illness, this chapter highlights the complex nature of lay people's views on expert systems. Giddens (1991a) questions the faith we place in expert systems; for instance, systems such as biomedicine. He argues that in a society faced by high levels of risk (nuclear war, environmental decay, AIDS), our faith in expert systems becomes limited. We no longer believe that they have the power to save us. Such limits propel us to search for alternative systems. In terms of health care, this can be seen to be a reason for people turning their backs on biomedicine and using alternatives. What the accounts of the women within this research show, however, is that while women do use alternative medicine, their faith ultimately still rests with the expert system of biomedicine. People still trust Western biomedicine to give them the answer to illness. This is something that will be explored further in Chapters 3 and 5.

This chapter also highlights the significant ways in which illness type intersects with social context. As the women's accounts show, health choices are not purely a response to health and illness, but are also informed by cultural and social resources. While the women were more likely to draw on particular types of non-Western or Western remedies for particular types of illnesses, their ability to do so depended on their social circumstances. As we can see within this chapter, while women's illnesses determine their health choices, these choices cannot be divorced from their geographical location or the strength of their social networks. For the women in this study, ethnicity also significantly influenced their responses to illness and their use of various remedies.

The fact that the women were part of a globally dispersed ethnic group as well as being British born widened their access to different and particular types of remedies. A person from a different background would respond to illness in a different way.

In demonstrating the significance of illness on respondents' health choices within this chapter I have begun to explore the importance of contextual circumstances on health choice. Family, generation, and life course also influence health choices. It is to these areas I will now turn.

NOTES

1. Bodily silence signifies a time when all feels well with the body and we do not think about it on a day-to-day basis. Bodily alienation or betrayal, on the other hand, signifies a bodily breakdown and shift toward illness. We become aware of our bodies when something goes wrong, and we feel betrayed by the body. These shifts and bodily interruptions have been written about within much of the literature on chronic illness, such as Bury (1982), Leder (1990), and S. J. Williams (1996, 2000).

2. See Bordo (1990) and Davis (1997) for wider debates on women and the body.

3. Hakims are practitioners of the Muslim medicine Unani, while Vaidas are practitioners of the Hindu medicine Ayurveda.

4. The overrepresentation of women and certain ethnic minority groups (e.g., Afro-Caribbeans) within statistics on mental health has been well documented (Pilgrim and Rogers 1993). Both groups are seen as being more likely to be diagnosed with problems associated with mental health. Debates around reasons behind this have been broad, with explanations ranging from methodological inaccuracy to labeling theory. For a fuller discussion of these debates, see Busfield (1996) for women and mental health and see Nazroo (1997) and Rack (1982) for race, ethnicity, and mental health.

5. Matthews and Larson (1997) chart the links between religion and medicine. By "prayer and Prozac" they are referring to the combined use of religion and medicine for (mental) illness. They portray a future where any divides between religion and medicine will be deconstructed. For a more detailed discussion of these links, see Chapter 4.

Chapter 3

Family, Generation, and the Life Course

This chapter addresses three areas central to the literature on women and health: family, generation, and the life course. Authors such as Blaxter and Paterson (1982), Charles and Walters (1998) and Graham (1993) have highlighted the importance of all three on women's health choices. Drawing on the family ties of women within the study, this chapter examines the way in which family, generation, and life course affect British Asian women's use of Western and non-Western remedies. In particular, there has been significant interest in the family and health literature on women's roles as mediators of family health. In capitalizing on this interest, the chapter explores women's gendered positioning within the family. It explores their roles as mothers and mediators of family health, and the ways in which they influence family use of syncretic medicine. The chapter also highlights the important intersection of ethnicity and family influence with geographical location. The women within this study are members of a globally dispersed ethnic group. Their family members are located in various parts of the globe. As will be shown, familial influence can be seen to work on local, national, and global levels.

WOMEN, HEALTH, AND THE FAMILY

There has been a significant amount of feminist research within sociology that has focused on women and health and illness (Doyal 1995). On both sides of the Atlantic research has highlighted the gender bias of the health profession, in terms of both research and practice (Bayne-Smith 1996; Kirchstein 1991). Studies have highlighted the tendencies within research to equate women's health purely with reproduction (Raftos, Mannix, and Jackson 1997). Research has also shown differences in men and women's health status, women's being in general significantly worse than men's (Blaxter 1990; Graham 1993). Broadly speaking, the belief held in developed countries suggests that women live longer than men but appear sicker and suffer more disability (Doyal 1995; Macintyre 1996). In assessing the gendered nature of health, researchers have also cast their gaze on the influence of marriage and cohabitation on the health status of men and women. Some research indicates that women's health behavior differs according to their marital status (Jones 1994; Popay and Jones 1990). As Arber (1997) argues, many studies of the 1970s and 1980s suggested that while marriage appears to be beneficial for a man's health it seems to be less beneficial for a woman's. However, Arber suggests that such patterns may no longer hold in light of recent changes in marriage patterns reflected in an increase in divorce rate and a growth in cohabitation. If we look at research on single mothers the picture appears bleak. Such research has highlighted how single mothers are more likely to have bad health than married or cohabiting mothers (Popay and Jones 1990).

More generally, research on family health focuses on the connection between women's activities as primary caregivers in the family and in society at large and as primary consumers of health care for themselves and others (Graham 1993). Women urge their loved ones to seek medical care, they make the doctor's appointments for their family members, and they purchase over-the-counter medicines for families' bathroom cabinets. Similarly, they are more likely than men to monitor the health status of extended family members, to become caretakers to the elderly, the infirm, and sick children. Many studies have concurred with this (Bowes and Domokos 1993; Stacey 1988), arguing that women can be counted as unpaid health workers. Finally, health research has attempted to explore the influence of family health choices on women's health choices. Taking a generational approach, studies have focused on looking at if (and, if so, how) ideas about health get passed on from generation to generation. This type of research has mostly been carried out between mothers and children (in particular, daughters). Studies have tended to suggest (Blaxter and Paterson 1982) that while mothers (like the rest of us) transmit health messages, their children do not necessarily absorb them. Instead, the learning process is mediated not through the family's health culture but more directly through experience.

All three bodies of women's and family health literature are pertinent here. However, these debates have yet to really explore the role of family influence on women's use of plural medicines. They also oversimplify issues regarding the role of the family and neglect the changing nature of this role. Studies on pluralism in both Asia and Britain have been couched in terms of wider social processes, and have not really explored the role of the family. Through the accounts of the women studied here, this chapter aims to explore the influence of the family on health choice. This chapter draws on the literature mentioned, but takes a more complex and dynamic approach. It highlights the complexity of familial influence on the respondents' health choices, recognizing that the influence is locally, nationally, and globally based.

First, the chapter will explore the influence of marriage on women's health choices. Within the study, the women's accounts show that while marriage might have a negative effect on women's health status, this is not necessarily the case for women's choices. Regarding health choices, marriage in most cases actually opens up new possibilities, as partners introduce women to different types of remedies previously unknown. This can be seen as beneficial and promotes a syncretic use of remedies. Conflict between women and their partners mostly occurs over children's health and choices of remedy. Women, however, maintain their position as gatekeepers of family health.

The chapter will also explore women's health choices regarding children's health. On the whole, although women might try different types of remedies for their children, ultimately they are most likely to resort to Western medicines. Within this section the differences between women's attitudes to younger and older children and health choices will be explored. I will move on to explore the role of generation on women's use of various remedies, looking at their own mothers' influence on their health choices and what they hope to pass on to their children. Rather than taking a straightforward generational approach, as other literature has, I will explore the convergence and conflict between gender and generation in women's use of different medicines. Family influence will also be situated within the context of the women's life course. Within the study, women's health choices were captured at a particular time (mothers with small children), and these choices as such will continue to change as the family does. Within this framework I will argue that women use different remedies at different times in the life course.

LIFTING THE VEIL ON MARRIAGE

Marriage is a significant point for the women within the study when discussing their health and health choices. All except one woman within the study were married (the one exception was divorced). In exploring the role of men and marriage, one must recognize the diversity of marriage and its meanings within the South Asian tradition (Bhopal 1999). For instance, for Hindus and Sikhs the importance of marriage is primarily based on a sacramental union, whereas for Muslims it is primarily a contractual union. While this is so, Bhopal (1999) argues there are significant similarities between the three groups in terms of relationship of individual to the family, the social and economic importance attached to marriage, the family structure, and the possibilities for mate selection, all of which are important. There is also a need to mention that one of the respondents was Catholic. For Catholics, matrimony is based on a contractual and sacramental union. Catholicism emphasizes the importance of marriage and family for the renewal of society (Knight 2000). Despite these religious differences between the women within the study, the commonality of the influence of marriage on health choices and general health seemed to override these differences.

Within the study, some women had moved from various other parts of Britain, such as from Birmingham, Blackburn, or London, to marry men in Leicester. Many of the women were also married to men from India or Pakistan, while others were married to British Asian men. Marital and family influences on women's health choices therefore needed to be explored along local, national, and global lines. Women also often still had family in India. As Menski (1999) argues, marriage of women from British South Asian diasporas transcends national boundaries, as many women marry men from India, East Africa, the Americas, and elsewhere. This demonstrates that Britain's ethnic minorities are today part of global social structures, and these in turn play a significant role in influencing health choices (see Chapter 5).

Arber (1997) has demonstrated the links between the institution of marriage and the differences in the health status of men and women. She concluded that while marriage is beneficial to men's health and mental well-being, it is hazardous to women. Women within this study felt that their general health altered as a result of marriage. As Samina's account shows, women saw marriage as having quite a negative effect on their health, involving more visits to the doctor:

Well I do tend to go more now for myself since I've been married because I can hardly remember going to the doctor for anything before I was married. I hardly ever used to get ill then, compared to now.

Within the research, women talked about the gendered division of labor between themselves and their husbands regarding their health status, suggesting men made more of a fuss of being ill then women. This was mostly said tongue in cheek and was compared to the women's own stoic attitudes toward health and illness. Inder's account highlights such differential attitudes often displayed by men and women:

> With my husband, I find that, if he's got a cold he's quicker than I am to get something from the chemist. He's always like "oh I'm dying," but we can both have exactly the same cold.

Many other studies have found similar results (Currer 1986). Cornwell (1984), for instance, in her study on working-class communities in East London, found that the gender division of labor impacted upon women's response to illness, in that while men could take time off work, women could not. As one respondent in her study notes,

> Men they're like babies. You don't know what I put up with from him. Women they get on with it. . . . I'd say women have more aches and pains than men but, as I say, when you've got a family you will find a woman will work until she's dropping. But she'll do what she's got to do and then she'll say, "Right, I'm off to bed." Whereas it is all-right for a man he's got nothing to do, he just lies there doesn't he? (p. 140)

This is related to the argument that women don't have the time to be ill, as they are the principal carers for the rest of the family (Charles and Walters 1998; Popay 1992). Women within this study felt that they were too busy to be ill. Gender divisions in attitude were also reflected in respondents' and their partners' consumption of public health care. In talking about visits to the doctors, while women in the study all went frequently, very few of their husbands did. Rambha's view of this was quite typical:

> My husband has been to the doctor's recently, to be honest he'd never been to a doctor's before. In fact the doc-

tor used to say, we don't see you that often, we hope to
see you once a year, just to make sure.

Again, many other studies that exemplify women's role as
caregivers within the family support this (Doyal 1995; Graham 1984,1993).

As shown, women's accounts emphasized a deterioration
in the overall quality of their health upon getting married.
However, the effects of marriage on women's actual health
choices was not quite so negative. Husbands clearly influenced women's use of Asian medical products and systems,
particularly when the husband came from India as an adult.
Men's influence on women's use of non-Western medicine
opened up a number of possibilities for women, enabling
them to try remedies on themselves and their families that
were previously unknown to them. This was seen in most
cases to be beneficial. Surinder, a Sikh woman from Birmingham, talked about how she had learned a lot about Asian
medical practices from her husband:

> His [her husband's family] are from India so there are
> other things that I've picked up from him. Like all kinds
> of remedies and things that I never knew before.

This highlights the significance of women's local–global
ties for their health choices. As British Asian women married to men from India, women's access to different types of
remedies opens up as national boundaries are transcended.
Such an influence of husbands on health choices occasionally even overrode the influence of respondents' mothers and
other members of the family. As Rabinder suggests,

> I only use mild herbal things. I wouldn't say that I've
> got them off my mother either, I'd say that I picked them
> up more in general, from my husband.

In the majority of cases within the study husbands would
tell their wives about various non-Western remedies, but there

was no pressure for women to use these. Respondents often use them in conjunction with Western remedies and health care as they see fit. As Rambha's account shows,

> Oh well he [her husband] tells me about all these differ-ent types of remedies from India and stuff. Sometimes I use them, other times I just go straight to the chemist but mostly I will try both.

For Samina, however, a Muslim woman married to a man from India, this encouragement to use non-Western medi-cine became somewhat forceful and ended up making her quite ill:

> My husband he's really into Indian remedies and things. I was suffering from hay fever about two weeks ago, badly, and I was gasping for breath and that's how bad I was. He said go and do this. There are these little seeds you get and they're really strong and I give them to him [her child] when he has asthma and his cough and ev-erything. I said to him [her husband] that won't help me 'cause it's for chesty things and he says just "take it." . . . I had to do it just to get him to keep his mouth shut and it made me really bad, I had to go to hospital.

For Samina, these differences in attitude reflected more gen-eral conflicts of identity between being born in Britain and being married to an Indian-born man. Such differences in this particular case also contributed to feelings of depression:

> I actually put up with a lot from him. I've adapted to his ways a lot so he should be doing the same for me you know. He just doesn't listen and it's hard.

This resulted in Samina going straight to Western medicine for solutions and comfort:

> I tried to get my husband to understand. I talked to my doctor permanently because I knew he would under-

stand and I felt that he could relate to me whereas my husband, he just couldn't because he's from back home. That's the only thing I can say because that's the only reason I can think of because we're not the same.

This negative effect of a husband's influence on his wife's health choices can be seen as an example of what Gardner (1990) sees as the social control of women. Men's influence on women's health choice and health in general helps to sustain the power of men and elders.

Within the research, men and marriage were influential on both women's health status and their health choices. Women in the study, however, talked little about their effects on men's overall health, although they were implicitly doing the majority of caring work for the men. They did, however, talk about their "lack" of influence on the choices men make about their health. What is interesting here is that men's friendship networks seemed in some ways to be more influential on men's health choice than women's influence. As Raminder pointed out,

My husband went to a healer, one of his friends told him about it, not me. He got some pain in his knee but it helped, it's all right now.

An area within the study where women and men's ideas about health clashed was over children. Men were often far more flexible about health care regarding women's health than they were with children. Men were quite cynical about women using Asian medical products and care on children and were often strongly against it. Zahira, a Muslim woman, discussed her husband's resistance to her using alternatives on their daughter:

No my husband's never let me use Asian remedies. If I wanted to do something that my mum did. No he wouldn't let me do that. He will say why are you doing things like this. Like the salt remedy my grandma told me about which gets inflammation down. He said no, it doesn't matter because only antibiotic medicine can help with that. I do them myself you know and he doesn't mind, for her he doesn't let me.

As this quote demonstrates, while the husband was resistant to her using alternatives on their daughter it was acceptable for her to use them on herself. However, despite men's cynicism, the ultimate decision on what to do about children's health was left to women. Shahnaz said,

He's like, oh aren't you taking them to the doctor's or have you taken them to the doctor but then I'd make the final decision as to whether its necessary to take them or not.

This again supports the literature on women's roles as caregivers and gatekeepers of family health. While men like to have a say in the decision-making process regarding children's health, ultimately it is women who are responsible for it. As Graham (1984, 1993) argues, as principal caregiver the mother acts not only as the home nurse, doctor, and tutor; she is also the person in contact with the professionals who perform these roles in the public domain. Typically it is the mother and wife who seeks out the health professionals for both husbands and children; she is the one who is also sought out by them.

Marriage and men can be seen to influence women's health choices, in particular their use of non-Western remedies. While in the general context of women's health marriage could often be seen to have negative effects, regarding actual health choice men's influence could in most cases (except for one) be seen to open up possibilities for women. Ultimately, marriage did not prevent women from using the remedies and medicine they wanted to, particularly regarding their own health. Women within the study acted on their desire to use non-Western and syncretic remedies (Rajan 1993). As such, it can be argued that respondents use various remedies in response to but also as part of a negotiation of gendered spaces within the private domain. Women assert and maintain their position as primary caregivers and gatekeepers of family health, as well as asserting their own health choices.

In-laws also influenced the women's health choices once the women were married. Influence was tempered by whether women lived with or close to in-laws. Many women, particularly Muslim women, lived with their in-laws after marriage. Accounts demonstrated how constraining in-laws could be on the women's lifestyles in general and specifically in relation to health choices. Many women were at odds with their in-laws and related this to their being from India. Samina, who moved in with a whole group of her husband's family after marriage, felt this:

> My in-laws when we were living together we would never see eye to eye because they're all from back home [India].

This in turn had negative effects on women's health. In the case of Samina, on moving in with her in-laws she became extremely depressed:

> I had him [her child] but I had a lot of pressures from my in-laws and my father-in-law and he quite often made me cry.

Other research has supported this argument about the difficulties women face after marriage when opinions of in-laws differ significantly from their own (Bhopal 1999). What was interesting within this research was that many women saw their in-laws as somehow more backward, particularly those from India, Pakistan, or East Africa. They often contrasted this to their own parents (though they were from India as well), who they felt were more forward looking. Respondents portrayed their own parents as more "Westernized." As will be shown in Chapter 5, these notions also intersect with national location, relating to where in-laws come from in Britain. In-laws who were based in northern cities within the United Kingdom, such as Blackburn, were often seen as more backward than those who lived in London or southern cities. Leicester was often placed somewhere in-between, termed by some as the "Asian village" because of its large South Asian population, while also recognized to be fairly cosmopolitan. This significance attached to the geographical location of in-laws highlights the importance of national geographical location on health choice. As Gurinder put it,

> All Asians are the same. Same crap. I think my in-laws are less Western than my parents, my parents are more Westernized. But the fact that they live in London, my parents. My in-laws came over here [from India] and settled in the north, that makes the difference.

This not only affected women's actual health status but also their health choices. They were not able to use the Asian remedies and products they might have used had they been at home with or close to their mothers. This was because women felt that in-laws and particularly mothers-in-law lacked knowledge about non-Western health practices. Shahnaz, a Muslim woman who had moved from Blackburn to London to Leicester, felt particularly constrained regarding the use of certain Asian remedies because her mother-in-law was not in favor of them and her own mother was in London:

> I think, to be honest, my parents used to be more into Asian remedies then my in-laws are here. You know I told you about remedies for things like bed wetting. I remember my mother used to make something for that and I asked my mother-in-law about that and she hadn't even heard of it.

This illustrates the important role the respondents' own mothers had on mediating their health choices (Blaxter and Paterson 1982). This again carried a spatial dimension;

women were prevented from carrying out certain alternative practices because they were reliant on their mothers' help and their mothers often resided in other places.

Within the study, women felt pressure from husbands to use certain remedies regarding their children's health, and in-laws put even more pressure on women. Women talked about how they felt as if in-laws thought they weren't looking after their children and their children's health needs properly. To go back to the example of Samina,

> My father-in-law, I was living with him. I was giving my baby bottle milk, what with all the demands of the household, housework and cooking, etc. it was too much pressure to breast-feed. Then he got colic and they [her husband's family] all thought it was something I was doing.

While respondents' experiences of in-laws were diverse, in-laws for the most part were seen to have a negative effect on women's health, particularly on women's emotional well-being. They also seemed to have a constraining effect on women's health choices, particularly regarding the use of Asian medicines and children's health. Such a directing influence over women, however, was only a temporally specific measure. Women lived with in-laws for a short period of time when married but then moved out to places of their own. While in-laws remained influential on women's health choices, they weren't quite as constraining. This is reflected in their choices and use of remedies as they moved into spaces of their own and become freed up regarding their health choices.

HEALTH CHOICES FOR CHILDREN

As already demonstrated in the first section, women are ultimately the principal carers within the family (Graham 1985, 1993), particularly of children (Blaxter and Paterson 1982). Women are not just mediators in children's health in terms of gaining appropriate professional care for their children and conducting activities directly related to health care procedures. Women also, through housework and cooking and cleaning are directly responsible for children's health (Graham 1985). Within the study some women were engaged in paid employment while others were not. Regardless, women were the ones taking primary responsibility for the health of their children on a day-to-day basis.

It can be argued that health can be seen to be a "moral category" when ascribed to the carer (Graham 1984). This relates to the argument of Radley and Billig (1996) that health accounts put forward by people actually signify their position in relation to the world and others and form a significant part of their identity. This has been reflected in health studies that focus on children. As Blaxter and Paterson (1982) argue in their study on mothers and daughters, women were reluctant to define their children as unhealthy, seeing it as a negative reflection on their mothering skills. The women within this study were initially reticent when talking about their children's health, readily defining children as healthy. As the interviews progressed and rapport was built, women talked more intimately about their children's health and ill-health.

Many women talked about their children's health in relation to their own. They noted how they were more likely to visit the doctor for their children's health. Rambha's response to the differential use of services for herself and her children was quite a common one:

> Myself, I try and wait for five days before I go to the doctor's because I tend to but with the children I never take the risk because you never can tell.

As we saw in the section on marriage, women in the study seemed to go to the doctor's more once they were married. This changed when they had children and become mothers. They went to the doctor's more for children's health and less for themselves. Women were also more likely to use private health care, such as the British United Provident Association (BUPA), for the children's health than for their own. Children's health became the focus of family concerns. As Surinder put it,

> I'd say that for the kids I have to go quite regularly [to the doctors], it used to be for me mostly but that was before the kids.

Regular use of the doctor for children was temporally specific and altered as children got older and as women had more children. Women's attitudes changed over the life course; in general, they became more relaxed. As Inder said,

> Children are such an experiment. My eldest daughter, I used to take her to the doctor a lot. After a while all I knew was that she got colds quite a lot. I just stopped taking her and kept her at home and used more things from home like honey and lemon.

Respondents also spoke on the subject of sex and gender of children. While the biological sex of the child was of importance to the wider family, women themselves did not mind whether they had male or female children. Women did not seem to treat the health of male and female children differently; they used the same remedies (whether Western or non-Western) on both and had the same attitude about GPs and practitioners of Asian medicine. Within this study, however, women did place gendered concepts of health and illness on boys and girls. Boys' health was perceived to be different from girls' in the sense that they would be more accident prone, as "boys will be boys." As Priya, a Hindu woman who has both a son and daughter, argued,

> Yes, he had stitches, here he fell off his bike and fractured his skull. It's the boys, they are rough, not like the girls.

While the women focused more on their children's health, their own health deteriorated upon having children. As Surinder shows, many women attributed this to lack of time to actually look after their own health because so much of their time was taken up by children:

> Just in general I could be doing a lot more for myself but I think it's really hard when you've got kids, it's hard to keep up. Running around after them. I want them to be well fed and well looked after and then I tend to forget myself and my own health.

As with marriage, the women showed that while having children might have negative effects on their health, their access to a plurality of remedies was not closed off upon having children. Because of the time constraints placed on women by children, women seemed to increase their own use of home remedies, both Asian and Western. Thus, children did not put constraints on women's use of syncretic remedies for themselves. They led rather to a shift of focus from women's public use of syncretic medicines to a greater use of medicine within the domestic sphere. What was particularly interesting to explore, though, through women's roles as carers and mediators, were women's attitudes to their children's use of alternative remedies.

There is evidence that, in general, alternative therapies are being employed by parents to help children with a range of chronic illnesses. For example, recent studies have reported that 11 percent of children attending a general pediatric outpatient clinic, 40 percent of children with cancer, and 70 percent of children with chronic juvenile arthritis used alternative therapies (Andrews et al. 1998). Other research on children and alternative health has come in the form of guidebooks to various alternative practices (Price and Parr 1996), or has focused on the influence of Western assimilation on migrant women's child-rearing practices (Gupta and Gupta 1985–1986). Within my study, while women's views on using Asian medical products or services for young children were quite mixed, some women did use some remedies. Women were quite keen to use herbal home remedies on the children. Charlotte, for instance, a Catholic woman, quite liked to use home remedies from the Caribbean on her children:

> I take ginger and massage their heads with oil. I do that with my kids, give them a good massage; it helps when they have headaches.

Women liked to use Asian balms, such as tiger balm, on their children for general ailments such as colds and flu. As Shahnaz, a Muslim respondent, observed,

> I like to use tiger balm on the kids quite often.

As argued in Chapter 2, these balms were readily available in Leicester. Some women within the research used these remedies on children because they felt they were milder and more natural and less risky than Western remedies. In this sense, their use of Asian medicines can be seen to fit in with the increase in the use of alternative medicine in general (West 1992). As much of the literature on alternative health demonstrates, many people are turning to alternative health care because of a disillusionment with Western health care and the much publicized long-term side effects of drug use (Worsley 1997). This is also linked implicitly to the wider debates concerning risk, health, and lifestyle (U. Beck 1992; Giddens 1991a; Turner 1991). Certain lifestyles are deemed to carry more health risk than others; for instance, the person who eats badly and does not get regular exercise increases the chance of suffering from heart disease (Nettleton 1995). As mentioned in Chapter 2 regarding risk and health, sometimes not even expert systems can be deemed to save us, which is why people now look to alternatives in a variety of realms. In talking about environmental risk, Giddens (1991a) exemplifies this well:

Widespread lay knowledge of modern risk environments leads to an awareness of the limits of expertise and forms one of the "public relations" problems that has to be faced by those who seek to sustain lay trust in expert systems. . . . Realization of the areas of ignorance which confront the experts themselves, as individual practitioners and in terms of overall fields of knowledge, may weaken or undermine that faith on the part of lay individuals. (pp. 130–131)

Women within the research generally liked to try alternatives on children because they perceived them in many ways as more natural and better for overall long-term health. Regarding asthma, many women talked about the use of non-Western remedies. Research has shown that a substantial proportion of children with asthma who attend pediatric clinics use alternative therapies (Andrews et al. 1998). Within the study, some women would try alternatives rather than have their children dependent on long-term use of inhalers or steroids. Inder's argument demonstrates:

My eldest daughter seems to be getting asthma. The doctor wants her to get an inhaler but I've said no. She's got some medication for the cough that she's got. But I've found that giving her hot rather than cold drinks helps and changing her bed linen everyday helps. I'd rather do that than her use an inhaler.

The women did quite often like to use Asian remedies because they seemed more "natural" than biomedical ones. Women did worry, though, if their children were already on medication with the GP. While women would continue to use Asian home remedies, they were quick to resort to Western medicine if non-Western remedies were not working. This was despite the risks involved. Ultimately, as argued in Chapter 2 regarding serious illness, the women had more confidence in the overall success of Western medicine. As Samina suggests,

Like I said he suffers from asthma and I've got to be careful with him, I've got to, I have to take him to the doctor. He's been in hospital once. I treat him at home with Asian remedies and then with him having asthma I have to take him to the doctor's.

This attitude did vary according to illness (see Chapter 2). Within the study, women also took their children to visit Hakims and Vaidas for various illnesses, such as asthma, diabetes, and eczema, which required long-term treatment, but quite often found that these clashed with treatments from GPs. Again, women were ultimately happier to stick with Western medicine, as Sakeena's trip to a hakim for her daughter's asthma demonstrates:

I took my daughter for eczema. What happened is they stopped her other doctor's medication for asthma, her inhaler. What happens if she has an attack? You know, these Hakims they treat from the root so they take a longer period and take a "holistic" approach. It enhances the illness then cures it. We didn't want to take the risk.

Hillier and Rahman (1996) reported similar findings in their study on parental perceptions of emotional and childhood development among Bangladeshis in East London. They showed that while the mullah and prayer played an important role in times of illness among children, GPs were the most favored source of help. It appeared in this study that while women were willing to use both Asian home remedies and practitioners for their children's health, they were happier using Asian home remedies than seeking out Asian medical practitioners. Women within the study did take their children to visit Hakims and Vaidas, but were more skeptical about this and ultimately would rather take them to the GP. Women differentiated between their own health and that of their children. As Pryia shows, on the whole, while it was acceptable for the women to use alternatives and Asian remedies, they were not as happy for the children to:

We take things like ginger and remedies; for me, I do this, for the children I go straight to the doctor. Because if I don't give the right medicine to the kids it's not good, for me it's less important.

This may reflect back on men's role in the decision-making process regarding children's health, even on the lay referral network. It also may in part be related to the imposition of biomedical models on the women by community health workers during the prenatal period (Karseras and Hopkins 1987). The findings support the argument that while women in the project still drew on syncretic remedies regarding children, they were less confident in doing so for the children than for themselves. While their position as British Asian women gives them access to a plurality of remedies, their gendered positioning within the family constrains their active seeking out of such remedies. There appeared less of a feeling of resistance to both their gendered positioning and to biomedicine. This emphasizes the significance of gender and ethnicity, both of which produce new possibilities as well as constraints on the women's health choices.

Teenage Resistance

In much of the literature, young people are seen to look more to peers than to parents for confirmation of maturing identity. Parents are seen to have a negative effect on adolescent identity, and adolescents will identify themselves in direct opposition to parental desires (Apter 1990). Research on adolescent health has demonstrated that, on the contrary, while conflicts do exist between young people and parents, parents and particularly mothers still have a significant role to play in mediating teenage health (Brannen, Dodd, Oakley, and Storey 1994). While young people begin to visit the GP unaccompanied, mothers are still seen to be active in recognizing signs of illness in their teenagers, helping them decide what to do, making GP appointments, and so on. This is seen to be particularly the case for daughters (Brannen et al. 1994). Husbands' roles regarding teenage health are viewed as becoming negligible.

A number of women in the study had eldest children who were teenagers. Women felt that regarding children aged up to about twelve, they had ultimate control and sanction over administering health decisions. Regarding teenage children, however, the women's role became much more contested. According to the respondents' accounts, it appeared that teenage children's health choices were far from syncretic. On the whole, teenage children felt the need to go to the doctor on a regular basis and would rather go to the doctor than try anything at home, Asian or otherwise. In talking about her teenage daughters, Raminder argued,

Oh my god they are fussy, always to the doctor.

Concurring with Brannen et al. (1994), women within the study still took a major role in making appointments and mediating with health professionals. However, women's suggestions about health were not always taken. Teenage children tended to be cynical about the use of Asian medical systems and would refuse them. On trying to get her children to use various Asian herbal remedies, Rambha argued,

I've tried that with the children and they're a bit skeptical. They wouldn't try this, they wouldn't touch it. They say are you sure this is all right. They would rather go to the doctor.

The women associated this with the impatience of adolescent culture. Teenagers often felt that they wanted a quick fix from the doctor and, as already argued, as Asian remedies and healers take a holistic approach to health, many practices take longer. Teenagers do not seem to have time for this. Sakeena found her teenage daughter particularly resistant to using Asian remedies and health practices:

Yes, but she is so uncooperative. Straightaway she goes to the doctor and she's so fussy. I've tried to get her into aromatherapy and things because she's so hyper but she won't listen.

This stands in opposition to other research on generational differences in health choices within families. In a study on the health and health behaviors of migrant South Asians and younger-generation (mostly British-born) Asians, R. Williams and Shams (1998) argue there are few differences in health choices between generations. They argue that this is the case despite pressures to conform to teenage norms. They relate this tentatively to factors in teenage socialization within British Asian families, seeing factors such as high levels of parental protection, religious beliefs, and the value placed on schoolwork as influential. At the very least, they suggest that this is an indication of the strength and vitality of British Asian cultures.

Overall, within the study women gave the impression that teenagers were happy for their mothers to continue to do informal health work for them and to continue to act as mediators with professionals. They were, however, resistant to women's suggestions that they use Asian medical practices and systems, and wanted to locate themselves completely within Western medicine. In the case of women with teenagers in this study, peer pressure seemed to take significant precedence over parental influence. Also, rather than taking an oppositional stance to dominant cultural forms, as youth culture has been traditionally viewed as doing since World War II, according to the mothers, teenagers located themselves firmly within Western consumer culture (Carter 1984). This could be linked to the overall identity of teenagers and may be temporally specific, altering as teenagers progress through the life course. Donovan (1986) argued in her study on South Asian and Afro-Caribbean women's health in London that some informants wanted to adopt more Western ideas in order to keep up with their children. However, the children's choices did not seem to affect women's use of syncretic remedies, and in turn women's use of syncretic remedies was not seen to be translated to the next generation. This highlights the significance of taking a generational approach to exploring health choice. The women's position as second-generation British Asian women played a significant role in influencing health choices. Whether and in what ways the women's children's choices will become syncretic as they get older is yet to be seen. These interactions and influences of generation on use of health remedies will be further explored in the next section.

FROM GENERATION TO GENERATION

As argued in Chapter 1, little research has focused on the influence of generation on the health choices of minorities and migrants. Taking what Goldberg (1993) calls an ethnic reductive approach, studies have failed to recognize the importance of generational specificity on health choices. Some studies on migrant and minority health have alluded to generational differences based on patterns of migration, length of settlement, and generational positioning (Kraut 1997). Studies have also explored the differences in general health between British-born and migrant generations, noting a general improvement over generations in health. This has been related to changes in health behaviors, focusing on issues such as diet (Williams and Shams 1998). However, research has yet to explore the impact of generation thoroughly, particularly in regard to its intersection with the life course. There are studies focusing on the impact of generation that are situated in significant moments in the life course. These studies have focused on looking at the influence of mothers on the health beliefs and behaviors of children (Blaxter and Paterson 1982; Campbell 1975b; Mechanic 1964). Such research has failed so far to make any kind of direct correlation, suggesting instead that a more informal learning process between women and children takes place. These studies have tended to focus on ethnically White and indigenous members of communities and countries.

One of the aims of this book has been to explore the influence of generation on health choice, in particular focusing on British Asian mothers; that is, Asian women who have lived in the United Kingdom for most or all of their lives. With this focus in mind, the influence of generation and its interactions with notions of length of settlement are explored. The temporal specificity of women's position within the life course is considered and there is a recognition that this position changes over time. Women within the study often talked about the importance of their own mothers' health choices and their influence on the respondents themselves. Many women's use of herbal and Asian remedies came from their mothers' usage. Women within the study trusted their mothers' judgment about alternatives, as Musarat, a Muslim woman, points out:

> Yes sometimes you have to go to the mother, they know what's better, they know this is a good cure. They've done it for years and it's been like a good cure. Even now, the use of balms and things I was telling you about, I learnt that from my mother.

In fact, some women felt that they would use non-Western care only if their mothers had recommended it. In talking about Chinese herbal remedies, Gurinder, a Sikh respondent, said,

> Only because my mum brought it and made it up. I wouldn't do it otherwise, wouldn't go off on my own and do it.

The women frequently felt that their general ideas about health were the same as their mothers. While health choices were perhaps not necessarily passed on from mothers in a direct, straightforward fashion, mothers' influence on health choice was far stronger than being a mere informal learning process. Women quite often seemed to take the same route in health-seeking behavior as their mothers, as Sakeena points out:

My mum and me do the same things regarding health.
First we use a remedy from home, if it's not working
then we go to the doctor.

Within the study, women felt very strongly about this and
often stated that their mothers' recommendations regarding
health and health care worked better than those of doctors.
Recommendations were strongest around issues of pregnancy,
as noted in the previous chapter, but mothers also gave advice about grandchildren that the women often heeded. As
Priya, a Hindu woman, argues,

Yes, with the children she [her mother] says like, use
certain types of herbal powders so we try that. Sometimes they don't work and we take them to the doctor.

While the women themselves were eager to learn new
health choices from their mothers, grandchildren (the women's
children) were even more resistant to grandma's advice than
they were to their own mother's. As Rambha, who has a teenage son and daughter, demonstrates,

My mother has tinned powder, a mix of herbs. She has
it once a week, as a precaution rather. It clears the stomach and gets rid of bugs. It's bitter, I've tried it on my
children and they say never again, no way, they'd rather
take paracetemol.

Blaxter and Paterson (1982) studied a group of mothers
and their married daughters who were themselves mothers.
Their data suggest that attitudes are not transmitted in any
simple way from generation to generation. Instead, Blaxter
and Paterson found that similar attitudes existed only when
and to the extent that the mothers and daughters shared experiences born of a common environment. This relates to
some of the findings within this study, not regarding attitudes, but related to active choices made about health. While
ideas about health seemed to translate from mothers to the

women, in some cases actual practices recommended by the mothers could not always be carried out because women were located in different geographical areas from their mothers. Again, this highlights the importance of geographical location on health choices. When the women's mothers were not geographically close, living within the same city, women were often prevented from using some Asian health practices. Some Asian remedies, particularly those of a spiritual nature, when practiced on children often required the involvement of the mother's mother, particularly those associated with practices against the evil eye (see Chapters 2 and 4). Shahnaz, a Muslim woman with two children, talked about how she would like to carry out some health practices associated with the evil eye but couldn't because her own mother lived in London:

> I would do rituals associated with the "evil eye" more often. I do try and do it but it's better if a grandparent does it, but my mum's in London.

The women were further constrained at times by the fact that their mothers were in India, which was even worse than their being in another part of the United Kingdom. This also put extra worry on respondents about their own mother's health, as Priya's account shows:

> My parents are in Africa and my husband's family is in Madagascar. [Do you miss them?] Yeah, mum and dad. Especially as mum is not feeling well. So I miss my mum.

Within the study it seemed that women's dislocation from their mothers on marriage acted as a constraint, particularly regarding the use of Asian medicine. This highlights the ways in which family influence on health choices becomes guided or constrained by geographical location. Women talked about the influence of their mother's health choices on their own health choices. They also, however, focused on generational influence on their state of health, again focusing particularly on mothers. Some women talked about this in terms of their mothers passing on a strong constitution of health to them. Harpreet argues,

> I've definitely got that from my mum I reckon. I mean, she had a hysterectomy recently and she was strong over all that, the only thing she didn't do was picking her things up. Women who have that operation don't do those things for a few weeks but not my mum. She's quite strong.

Inder spoke in terms of generational fears of particular illnesses:

> I was actually worried, my mum had cancer. She had chemotherapy and everything and she's better now. I thought, if she's got it I'll get it and my children will get it. Now I know that's not necessarily the case, that there are other factors involved.

Grandparents and other relations, such as aunts and uncles, also seemed to have a role to play in influencing women's health choices. This came mostly from grandmothers and was particularly focused on the issue of advising women about herbal home remedies. While influential, though, grandmothers' influence on health choices on a day-to-day basis was limited. Some women's grandmothers had passed away and others lived in India. In the latter case women were often dependent on visits to India to gain any new advice. This did not stop women ultimately from using remedies passed on to them, and in fact gave them links to an "imagined homeland," as both Sita and Charlotte point out:[1]

> Again it goes back to my roots. Like you know I was very close to my grandma and she was my heroine really. I would take all kinds of things from her.

> My grandma used to make bush tea for health, so I have that.

Teenage resistance to their mother's health choices is something already explored in the section on children. This resistance did not prevent women from talking about ideas they would like to pass on to their children, as their own mothers did, and did not stop them from worrying about illnesses they might pass on. The last question in the interview schedule was based around ideas of what the women felt they would pass on to their children, in order to look at whether women thought that syncretic views would hold with the next generation. Women did talk about how they would like to pass things on to their children, particularly to their daughters. This was related to both Western and non-Western remedies. Sakeena, whose teenage daughter had shown so much disdain for her mother's "alternative" health choices, was keen to try and pass on some of her ideas:

> Actually, I wanted her to know and prepare when she goes away [to university]. She should prepare a folder of what to do when. Please I ask her, and she says mummy prepare it and give it to me.

Ultimately, though, women within the study emphasized the importance of the doctor to their children. Women wanted to point out that, ultimately, GPs know best. Rhamba said,

> Well, I wouldn't mind explaining to them the basics and tell them that some of these natural cures would work. Like inhaling mint that you have grown in the garden and just steam. That will help you breathe properly, if they've got a cold or something but I would also tell them that look, if you find that you're not better, have it checked out, never take that risk.

Overall, generation seemed to play a pivotal role in the women's accounts regarding family health choices. Mothers' influence on the women's use of particular remedies was significant and seemed to heighten their use of syncretic remedies. It did seem that women were drawing on their mothers' health choices more since they had became mothers themselves. In this sense, many women did talk about resistance to parent culture when they were teenagers, locating themselves more within Western culture. This changed upon marriage, when women's views became more syncretically located as they took on more ideas from parent culture. This highlights the ways in which the women's position as British Asians intersects with the women's position in the life course, recognizing that women's health choices change over the life course. Drawing on some of these issues, family influence will be explored within the context of the life course.

The Life Course, Generation, and Health Choices

In exploring women's health, Raftos, Mannix, and Jackson (1997) emphasize the multiple points within women's life course and argue that it is important to recognize that there are differences between these points in terms of women's health. In their study on ethnicity and identity, Woollett, Marshall, Nicolson, and Dosanjh-Matwala (1994) argue that one must recognize the ways identity changes over time during the life course. Focusing on a study of Asian women in London, Woollett et al. argue that women's identity is an ongoing process, changing developmentally in terms of transitions in women's lives as they marry and become mothers. Identity also changes as children grow up and go to school. Such a processual life-course approach to identity can be translated in this study to generational influence on health.

While recognizing that respondent's choices were reflective of a specific period in their lives, it was interesting to see that throughout the research women seemed to reflect on family health choices in both the past and future in terms of life changes they had gone through. Generation and the life course seemed to intersect, influencing women's health choices, as did length of generational settlement. Health choices change with each successive generation, becoming more socialized within British culture, and as women's life circumstances themselves change. The women's mothers' health choices changed over time, through length of settlement and progression through the life course. This was often reflected by a decrease in respondents' use of Asian remedies, as Rambha argues:

> Originally my mum used a lot of balm and herbs that came from India, but less so over time. I don't tend to use them a lot.

The women also recognized the changes in their own health choices as they progressed through the life course. Gurinder referred to a change in health choices upon getting married and getting older, being more likely to use alternatives as she got older:

> A few years ago I would have thought no need. You need hospital, a doctor, whatever. Over the years I don't think the same thing. I think I would seek alternative medicine. I would pass that on to my children too. I wouldn't mind trying what my mum's tried, some herbal remedies and stuff you know. I would try some of the things my mum did.

The health choices of the women's children were also temporally specific. Women felt that even children were most likely to take on some of their ideas when they became older and took on the role of parents. As Sakeena says,

> OK, if I leave all these things, if I tell her this, she will follow them when she comes into the role of mother you know. At this age seventeen, they hate their mother but you don't realize how much like their mother they are until they become a mother.

The influence on teenagers' health choices on their position as younger-generation women remains unknown. The trend toward their current affiliation with Westernization may be transcended when they reach adulthood, particularly when they become parents themselves. Perhaps there is the potential for their health choices to become syncretic then, but this may not be in the same way as their mothers' health choices are syncretic now. As Gilroy (1993, 3) argues with regard to Black British cultures, styles and forms of the Caribbean, United States, and Africa have been reworked and reinscribed syncretically in the context of modern Britain. One could argue that such syncretic styles and forms are reinscribed in a different way in other times and contexts. Ultimately, influence of generation was very important to the women and they would like to see things being passed on from generation to generation. Such a tradition is, however, also couched in notions of choice and time, particularly where their children are concerned. As Raminder argues in reflecting on passing health choices onto her children,

> It's about time, how do I know what I will tell my children. I believe that I don't want to force them into certain things. They have to make choices themselves.

Within this study, women do seem to have a clear sense of the impact of change, both generationally and as they progress throughout the life course and are faced by different stresses and strains. It appeared that the women's mothers' use of Asian remedies decreased, while their's were syncretic and their children's were mostly Western. This emphasized women's position under their current place within the life course and as British Asian women, socialized within the West but with parents who were migrants themselves. Family and generation affect women's health choices differently at differing times as women move throughout the life course.

Charles and Walters (1998), in their study of the health accounts of women of different ages in South Wales, emphasized the importance of women's position in the life course with regard to their health. Women's accounts demonstrate that their experiences and explanations of health, while showing certain commonalities, vary with age and stage in the life cycle and are shaped by wider structural changes in employment patterns and gendered division of labor. Thus, structural and cultural changes shape the remedies that women drew upon when talking about health and illness and help explain the similarities and differences in ways of talking about health between women of different generations. This study supports their argument within the context of syncrecy. Within the study, family and generation influence women's health choices. These must also be situated within the women's life course. However, as I will go on to show in later chapters, there are broader influences at work here. Other contextual circumstances intersect with these to influence women's health choices.

CONCLUSION

The influence of family, generation, and the life course on health choices has been the focus of this chapter. The chapter has highlighted the gendered nature of marital influence on women's health choices. Marriage has often been eclipsed within much recent research on gender and health. Rapid social change has been seen as the reason for such an eclipse. Drawing on data from the study, I have shown that marriage matters. As the findings of the research show, men still have a significant effect on women's health status, their sense of well-being, their stress, and their health choices. The research has been based only on interviews with women and therefore it is difficult to gauge the effects of marriage on men's health. However, according to the women within the research, by and large marriage seemed to have a beneficial effect on men's health. This highlights the ways in which influences on health choices are gendered. The chapter has also highlighted the ways in which health choices made on behalf of children's health are ascribed a moral status. Parents want to be seen to do the "right thing" for their children's health. The choices made for children's health are therefore complex; on the one hand, alternative remedies are deemed more natural, and on the other Western medicine is seen as best. This supports the argument made in the previous chapter that despite the increased use of alternative medicine our faith ultimately lies within the expert system of biomedicine.

This chapter has shown the ways in which health choices vary according to generation and the life course, thus highlighting the importance of ethnicity and generation. Age, stage of life, and length of settlement of migrant groups play significant roles. We see this in the women's accounts through the ways in which teenage children are much more keen to locate their choices within Western medicine. This stands in comparison to the women's parents, whose choices are more located with non-Western medicine. Overall, the accounts of the respondents highlight the complex interweaving of contextual circumstances with the women's position as British Asians. Such an intersection can be seen to contribute to respondents' syncretic health choices. Thus, the family plays a significant role in influencing women's use of remedies for themselves and others. Within this chapter I have shown the ways in which such familial influence intersects with local, national, and global contexts. From the women's accounts it is clear that the influence of family is both enhanced and constrained by geography. The influence of geographical location is something I will explore in more detail in Chapter 5. While women's syncretic use of remedies is significantly influenced by illness and by the family, they are also influenced by respondents' religion and community. These contextual circumstances also intersect with broader issues of identity. The influence of religion and community within the context of identity will be explored in the next chapter.

NOTE

1. "Imagined homeland" here is a play on B. Anderson's (1991) ideas of imagined communities. Anderson talks of the nation as an imagined political community. He sees it as imagined because the members of even small nations will never know of their fellow members, meet them, or hear them. However, according to Ander-

son, in the minds of each lives the image of communion. Drawing on Anderson, imagined homeland within this research is used to denote, in a spatial context, the women's relationships to India or Africa. They may never have lived in these places (or have any intention of doing so), or visit them that frequently, or know many people there. However, in the minds of many respondents these places still maintain the quality of mythical homelands.

Chapter 4

Religion, Community, and Identity

The previous chapter explored the influence of the women's families, generations, and lifestyles on their health choices. This emphasized the significance of women's ethnic group ties and the influence of social and geographical context on their health choices. This chapter continues to focus on the importance of ethnicity and context. Drawing on data from the study, this chapter explores the influence of religion and community on the women's health choices. The intersections between these influences will also be explored within the context of health and identity. In exploring such intersections of influence, the chapter highlights the difficulty of seeing religion or community as homogenous entities, as they are often portrayed within research. Rather, the chapter highlights the diversity within the categories of religion and community, emphasizing the multiplicity of their influence on health choices. Furthermore, through explorations of religion, community, and identity in the women's accounts, the chapter highlights the ways in which the influence of gender, generation, and ethnicity on health choices cannot be seen as fixed categories. Such categories are shown to be fluid in their influence, shifting over time and context.

Porter and Hinnells (1999) argue that the intersection between religion and health is universal throughout recorded history. They meet at the great turning points of life: at birth, at moments of acute suffering, and at death. Religion is far more than a mere set of beliefs or an optional way of life; it is also a conditioning, a powerful expression of identity, the embodiment of a received tradition of world views, of personal understanding, of values, priorities, hopes, and fears. Religion can be seen to influence the maintenance of good health. Marks and Hilder (1997) look at the influence of religious practices on health status. They look at low levels of infant mortality rates among Jewish children at the turn of the century. The stress that Jewish teachings placed on personal hygiene, cleanliness, and rituals associated with kosher food helped prevent food contamination and illnesses such as diarrhea. Within studies on health choices, religion is also often explored in its therapeutic capacities. Singh (1999) points to the positive effects of Sikh prayers on stress-related illness. Both in terms of health status and health choices, religion is often seen as a significant influence.

The term "community" has been used and explored in studies on health and on race and ethnicity. Its conceptualization remains open to a wide and diverse range of meanings, imaginings, and competing definitions (Crow and Allan 1994). Within discourses on health alone the term has been used in a dual context. It is used both as a shorthand term for services and organizations that are locally based and organized and as an ideology conveying notions of accessibility, local autonomy, responsiveness, social solidarity, and shared benefits (Jones 1994). If we expand the term "community" further the range of meanings is wider still: It may refer to groups with common interests, values, beliefs, or experiences on whatever scale they operate, both spatially and nonspatially (Jeffers, Hoggett, and Harrison 1996). Hahlo (1998) talks of community as consisting of a wide range of social exchanges between members. Taken as a whole this leads to a view of community as a socially constructed reservoir of scarce resources. This includes the maintenance of ties be-

tween groups based on marriage and allows for the maintenance of cultural and social values and attitudes, structures
of political support, and a range of social relations, including kinship and friendship (Hahlo 1998). On the whole, projections of community have created the illusion of fixity and
absolute identification. In talking about the Black community Alexander (1996) argues for more fluid and layered notions of community. Drawing on the findings of her study among
Black male youth in South London, she argues that community
exists on a variety of levels and the individual's reaction to it
can be seen to be multilayered and multifaceted.

Within this study, both religion and community influenced
respondents' health choices. Earlier chapters of the book have
already highlighted some of the ways religion influenced
women's health choices; for instance, in exploring illness
itself (Chapter 2). Within the current chapter I show how
religion informed women's use of particular types of remedies. While women within the study talked less about religion as a source of comfort, religion held a general influence.
Differences in health choices appeared according to women's
religions. This signifies not a difference in syncretic use of
medicine but in the type of non-Western remedies used. Community also influenced women's health choices, working on
a number of levels, from religious community through to
broader identifications with Asian communities and spatially
located communities. Women's accounts emphasized the intersecting influence from differing levels of community on their
use of particular types of remedies, both Western and non-
Western. Taken as a whole this multiple layered influence
led to an overall move to women's use of syncretic remedies.

The influence of religion and community are situated in a
temporal context, with religion influencing health choices
at particular times, and the broader community at others.
These influences also tie in with issues relating to identity
and health. A number of studies have focused on the relationship between health and identity. As shown earlier,
Radley and Billig (1996) argue that people's accounts of health
and illness are more than views about what people in soci-

ety should do to avoid disease; they also articulate a person's situation in the world and indeed articulate that world in which the individual will be accountable to others. When women within the study talked about health and illness they also talked in more general terms about their identities and their situations within the world. Through their accounts the women discussed their position as British Asians. Respondents' health choices often reflected their syncretic identity. Different aspects relating to women's identity, such as religion, community, and family (see Chapter 3), became more prevalent at particular times, as did their influence on health choices.

Within this chapter the influence of religion and community on health choices will be explored. This exploration will be related to more general issues of identity. As in previous chapters, accounts from the women in the study highlight the usefulness of the framework of syncrecy. In particular, the women's accounts highlight the uses of syncrecy in contrast to approaches that suggest this generation of migrant children are caught "between two cultures," both West and non-West. The accounts highlight the complexity of the respondents' positions, emphasizing the significance of contextual circumstances on syncretic use of remedies. Unlike previous studies, the accounts of the women researched here highlight the need to recognize the intersections between contextual categories such as community, religion, identity, and health, situating these within a dynamic temporal framework.

"WE'RE IN IT THE SPIRITUAL WAY": RELIGION AND HEALTH

Several women within the study discussed the importance of their religion and the general influence of religion on health. Women often felt that religion had a general role to play in good health and felt a connection between their spirituality and health. As Samina suggests, women frequently felt that they approached health issues in a spiritual way:

We [Muslims] believe in spiritual healers, we're in it the spiritual way.

While respondents talked in more general terms about the influence of religion on health, they also often used religious metaphors to signify their health. This is exemplified in an account from Charlotte, a Catholic respondent. She talks about the body as a "temple":

Your body is a temple and how you look after that temple is what you get out of it. If you let a lot of rubbish go into that temple, that temple will deteriorate and be destroyed, but if you look after that, your body as a place to worship, somewhere to clean, somewhere to respect, not to abuse, I believe you should look after that.

Overall, it was quite common for the women within the study to make general connections with health and religion at some level. Religion often acted as a general guideline to their health choices. This is something that has been common in previous studies on health choices. Religion was an important influence on the health behaviors of diabetes sufferers in Kelleher and Islam's (1996) study of Bangladeshi Muslims in Tower Hamlets. Religious ritual and festivals directly informed their diet. Authority of the doctor came second to the authority of God; for some, fasting included not taking tablets for diabetes. Religion was also influential in Donovan's (1986) study, with her respondents drawing on religion for issues of general illness.

In looking at the influence of religion on respondents' health choices, we can see a distinction between women of differing religions and their use of particular types of remedies. In relating to syncrecy, this was not to say, for instance, that Muslim women's health choices were syncretic but Hindu and Sikh women's were not. Rather, religious differences were highlighted within the women's accounts regarding the extent of religious influence, influence on public health care consumption, and types of remedy used. Muslim women seemed to draw on religion much more than Hindu and Sikh women, who used religion much more as a general frame of reference. If we refer back to the religious differences in Chapter 2 relating to certain types of illness, we saw how Muslim women drew very heavily on religion during pregnancy and for mental health problems. While Muslim women were very specific about eating hot or cold foods at particular points in pregnancy, Hindu women were much more concerned about associated religious traits and their impact on health. This exemplifies the split in the extent to which religion is drawn on. If we look at this statement from Samina, a Muslim respondent, we can see clearly the significance of religion, particularly surrounding issues of pregnancy:

> Yes, I draw on my religion a lot for health. It is particularly influential during pregnancy, in terms of food, prayer and everything. It means a lot.

Samina's words can be held in contrast to some of those in Chapter 3 from Hindu women, who seemed to draw on religion less and in differing ways. As Rambha shows,

> Yeah I'm Hindu, and I am a vegetarian. My whole family is, and it does make a difference. When I was pregnant for the first or second time, I can't remember which one I was told that I was low on iron, very anaemic and no matter how many iron capsules they gave me it didn't work, mum told me I had to drink ribena.

As well as varying according to the extent of influence, there were also religious differences in women's accounts relating to their consumption of public health care. There seemed to be much more of a concern within the Muslim women's accounts surrounding the sex and religion of a doctor. This related to respondents' use of health care for gynecological and obstetric issues. For instance, this is apparent if we look at Samina's account. She cannot visit her local GP for gynecological issues because he is the same religion and it would not be right for him to see her unclothed:

> Yeah, I like to have a woman doctor. Just the other day, well a couple of months ago, I had to have the coil fitted. My doctor's Asian as well as he's Muslim that means we are the same religion and I don't want to open my legs to him and say put a coil in. I had to ring St. Peter's clinic and arrange something there you know with a female doctor [both laugh], could be Asian could be White, don't mind as long as she's female.

This view was supported by a number of the Muslim respondents. However, Hindu and Sikh women within the study were much less concerned with the sex and religion of their doctors. Although some preferred an Asian doctor, few worried about the religion of the doctor, and while gender was at times an issue, with women in the study preferring to consult women doctors over gynecological issues, attitudes on the whole were far more relaxed, as Sita, a Hindu woman, shows:

> [Do you prefer to have an Asian GP or don't you mind?] Oh, I'm not bothered about that. [Do you prefer a woman doctor?] Sometimes, but I don't mind. It's good with my practice because there are equal amounts of men and women so you can see whoever.

Respondents' health choices also varied across religion in relation to the type of religious remedies used. Eade (1997) highlights the diversity among religious health remedies in his research on Muslim Bangladeshis in Tower Hamlets. As well as biomedicine, he identifies Islamic models based on Unani, teachings grounded in the Quran and the Hadith, and subsequent authoritative texts. He also identifies folk systems located in syncretic customs, often (but not exclusively) based on magic or sorcery. These systems are not seen to be bounded; models can be presented as different for analytical purposes. This is not necessarily the case in lay accounts, where they may not be so separate.

Several Muslim women within the study talked in particular about notions of the evil eye and utilized practices surrounding that. Notions of the evil eye and spiritual possession can be found in most cultures throughout history (Worsley 1997). In talking about Southern Italian immigration to the United States at the turn of the century, Kraut (1997) talks about the predominance of beliefs about the influence on illness of one who had the *jettatura* or *mal occhto* (evil eye), a belief that had no basis in the Roman Catholic theology and which the church succeeded in supplanting (p. 235). Within my research, while Hindu and Sikh women alluded to various practices associated with supernatural forces, it was mostly Muslim women who talked about this in a specific health context. This was often specifically but not exclusively in relation to issues associated with mental health, such as anxiety and depression. Illness attributed to the evil eye can be caused by a number of things and there are believed to be certain tests that can be done to see if illness is caused by the evil eye or not, as Shahnaz demonstrates:

> Like I said if a child has a fever I mean, my sister the first thing she would do is a little ritual to see if its an actual illness or whether it's just someone giving them the evil eye. . . . You know children if they catch someone's attention. If they like, you know [pause], just being jealous of someone not in a nice way, that can cause illness.

Shahnaz went on to talk about the rituals to tell if something is caused by the evil eye or whether it is real illness. If something is caused by the evil eye this particular ritual will get rid of it:

> She [her mum] just says these prayers then what they do is they get these salts. There are quite a few variations on it but she usually gets a handful of salt and

then while she says the prayer she circles the body of whoever she's doing and then at the end of it she puts it in a cup of water and they say you know it helps, 'cause you know salts are supposed to do the opposite and that will tell you the implication for what it is, if it's just a normal illness or something brought on by the evil eye.

This can be applied to many illnesses, not just mental illness:

My husband had irritable bowel syndrome so we suggested that he might just have the evil eye, so my mother-in-law's sister was actually here at the time and so he got her to do it on him. She did it and has said that somebody had been giving him the eye but it wasn't that which was causing his pain, it wasn't to that extent that it was causing him to feel bad.

In light of the illness not being caused by the evil eye, Shahnaz's husband then consulted a biomedical doctor, exemplifying a use over time of syncretic remedies. Kraut (1997) notes the temporally located nature of ideas relating to the evil eye. He focuses on Italian immigrants to the United States during the turn of the twentieth century. He argues the relationship of Italian immigrants and their children to modern medicine did not remain stagnant; customs, traditions, and beliefs altered with each succeeding generation raised in the United States. There were differences between younger and older generations. At times traditional beliefs associated with the evil eye as the cause of illness still found expression among all generations, but such beliefs were not pervasive and their prevalence was linked to an individual's class position. Within this study some women engaged in behaviors surrounding the evil eye. Women also drew on other non-Western and Western remedies, reflecting syncrecy in health choices.

The argument put forward by Kraut (1997), perhaps unwittingly, seems to suggest an argument of assimilation: The younger the generation and the longer the length of migrant settlement, the more Westernized health choices will be. This type of approach seems to suggest a process of assimilation among this generation's health choices, with a starting point of non-Western choices and an end point of Westernization. The women's accounts show this was certainly not the case within my study. The respondents' accounts highlight their syncretic use of remedies. This does not mean they were between two types of medicine, but rather held medicines in tension, favoring one or the other at different points in time. They did not slowly progress from one type of medicine to another in a linear fashion as time progressed. As argued previously, health choices reflected respondents' generational position and their position as British Asians. These health choices also changed over time according to illness type and as women progressed throughout the life course. This was not in any sense through becoming "more assimilated." Rather, many respondents felt they would draw on non-Western remedies more as they got older.

Religion held a general significance for most women within the study. It influenced all of the respondents' health choices to some extent. There were differences between women of varying religions and their use of particular remedies, with Muslim women drawing more directly on religion than Hindu and Sikh women. This does not suggest that the health choices by Muslim women were more syncretic than the others; rather it draws our attention to different types of syncrecy and diversity within non-Western or religious systems themselves. As argued by Porter and Hinnells (1999), religious systems themselves are far from internally coherent. Women draw on different types of non-Western remedies, not just those associated with religion. As we have seen in previous chapters, different remedies become prevalent for the women at different times and in differing contexts, changing as they move through the life course. Certain categories, such as religion or community, are influential at particular times and in differing contexts. As shall be shown, these come to reflect the differing layers of women's identity.

LAYERS OF COMMUNITY

Respondents' health choices were also influenced by community. As argued in the introduction to this chapter, community remains a contested term and has come to mean a number of things. As Jeffers, Hoggett, and Harrison (1996) argue, the term community denotes social groupings bound together by either shared identity or shared interests or both. Specifically, a community appears to be bound by a shared idea of what its members have and how they differ from others. Its members may have in common a shared sense of belonging to a particular spatial area, in which case we may think of the existence of the spatial community. Alternatively, a group may find unity in the sharing of culture, religion, lifestyle, or other characteristics.

Taking these different types of community into account, we can see the multiple levels upon which community operates. Within the women's accounts, community worked on a number of levels. The women most significantly talked about the influence of religious community and the influence of the more general Asian community. Alongside this they talked about socializing across different communities, both Asian and White, and the influence of this socialization on health choices. Within the study, women identified their position as British Asians, as women of a particular generational and ethnic group, as situating them in a particular way in relation to community. Through this positioning respondents were not "caught between" differing community types but moved in and out of them. This was reflected in influences on the respondents' health choices: Differing layers of community affected the women's use of different types of remedies, marking an overall syncretic effect. Within this section I will take each layer in turn to explore their overall effect.

In Chapter 3 I explored the significance of older generations within the family context and how they influenced women's health choices. Women in the study also drew advice from older women within their religious communities.

Musarat highlights the important influence of these elders on her use of non-Western medicine:

> Yes, sometimes you go to the community members, particularly elders. They know what's better, they know this is a good cure. Now the Vicks thing I told you about earlier, I learned that from a community elder.

In this sense, community influence can be seen to be an extension of family influence. The community elders of the women within the study were particularly influential in relation to gynecological and obstetric issues; again, this was particularly focused around use of non-Western remedies, as Jameela points out:

> Another thing old ladies from the community tell you is when you are in the later stages of pregnancy, you should eat hot foods. That means foods that are, you know, hot and slippery.

While the women frequently drew on their religious community, they also quite often found community to be quite constraining and so influence tended to be sporadic. Inder shows how constraining religious community can be. Inder works in a Sikh community center and our interview took place there. This was of great concern to other members of the community, and highlights some of the constraints placed by community on women:

> I mean here now. They'll not say, "Oh she's got someone with her" [meaning myself and Inder in Inder's office]. They will still come in wanting to know a) what are you doing here, b) what are you saying to me [both laugh]. But they want to know all the bits and bobs, what's going on. They're nosy, let's give them something to talk about!

The women's accounts highlighted a diversity within religious communities, and women often distinguished between generations within the community (like with family). Respondents recognized that there was generational change and they felt more at home with members of younger generations. Women within the study identified changes over time with each different generation and identified feelings of insularity with older generations. This is demonstrated in another quote from Inder:

> But with this generation it's changing. Well in the [community] center itself we've got an elderly center, an under fives, a disabled group and other activities. It can be very hard at times. I find that people that have been born here [United Kingdom] or like our [my and her] age [mid–late twenties] are O.K. to talk to, you know, but the ones who have actually been born in India or wherever they've come from, they've been brought up in those countries and they're different.

Within women's religious communities, while elders were useful for advice on issues such as health, British-born members were much easier to socialize with although these did not seem to have a direct influence on health choices. Respondents' socialization across second-generation women of other religions seemed more significant in terms of influence on health choices. This highlights the multiple layering of community and the many levels of influence on health choices. While community elders' advice was influential (particularly surrounding pregnancy), women also looked to the broader Asian community for general health concerns. Several women within the study socialized regularly with Asian women of other religions. Respondents' health choices in turn were often influenced by women of other religions. Most of the women within the study had Asian friends from other religious communities, as Sita, a Hindu woman, points out:

> I mix with all types of people here [at the center]. We have a couple of Muslim ladies, a couple of Punjabis,

Gujarati, we just mix in fact, and a lot of my best friends are Muslim girls.

Harpreet, a Sikh respondent, acknowledged conflict across religion as an important historical component of religious history. However, as with many of the other women in the study, she did not let this stop her from mixing across communities:

Yeah, a lot of people say that we're not supposed to mix with Muslims because of what happened a long time ago, and what happened with our Gods and all that, but you can't take that out on anybody.

This socializing across religions often influenced respondents' use of non-Western remedies. Through making friends with other women, women within the study learned and tried new non-Western remedies. This often went alongside the influence of women's own religions, as Sakeena, a Muslim woman, points out:

I have built up quite a social group of women who are Hindu and Sikh. I learn so much from them. They tell me all sorts of remedies specific to their religions and I try them. Some I use regularly. My own religion is also very influential on my health choices. There are so many remedies I have learned from my mum, and, yes, they are specific to the Muslim faith.

This influence was also extended to giving advice on various Western remedies.

My Hindu and Sikh friends will also tell me about Western remedies that I hadn't heard of before, they'll say "Oh have you tried such and such from the chemists for coughs?"

Within the study, women's friendships with women of other religions can thus be seen to be quite substantial and influence women's syncretic use of remedies.

This socialization across religions can also be seen in respondents' position within the wider "Asian" community. Women within the study at times talked in terms of their religious communities and about socializing with other religious communities; at other times they talked much more generally about being part of an Asian community. Ballard (1994) argues that to talk of an Asian community is often to reinforce a fiction. He highlights diversity among South Asian populations within Britain and argues that any meaningful solidarity between groups must be grounded in active networks. "Real" communities in his terms are much more parochially organized. Women within this study did talk about an Asian community, and as Espiritu (1992) in her work on Asian Americans argues, this community ranged from localized affiliations to a larger pan-Asian affiliation. The Asian community for respondents within this study was made up of people with Asian backgrounds of various religions. Within the research, this sense of community was both "real" in the sense that Ballard (1994) suggests, being locally contextualized, and also "real" and "imagined" in a more global context. This draws on Anderson's (1991) arguments about "imagined communities" (see Chapter 3), with connections between the Asian diaspora in various contexts at a face-to-face level remaining mostly within an "imaginary" realm. However, through the globalization process, with its emphasis on the deconstruction of borders and boundaries, respondents' visits to Asia and the Asian diaspora in other contexts enabled connections to become "real" at certain times. This will be explored in more detail in Chapter 5.

This section of the book focuses on the influence of the Asian community in its localized context. Women within the study talked in quite holistic terms about this community and would compare health choices of the community with those of "White" community members. Gurinder talked about how all communities have their folk remedies, Asian communities being no different:

Asian communities have the same sort of old wives' tales and things as Western culture you know, try this remedy or that. If you have a bruise put a chapati or something cold on it. Basically, you know, we have the same sorts of remedies, but I'm one of these people that, you know, I'm not going to say oh you shouldn't do this or you shouldn't do that but, if I think it will work I will have a go.

In this sense the Asian community influence was connected to use of folk remedies and advice from older members of the community. Respondents also talked about the Asian community and health care in much more general terms. For instance, some women talked about the inefficiency of "community" in a health care setting. Sakeena, for example, felt that treatment from the community within a health care center was bad:

It's experience, if "your" [Asian community] people are not very helpful. Sometimes you feel that White people are doing the job better and I'm sorry to say that, but this is the way.

When women within the study talked about an Asian community, they also emphasized that the nature of the community was changing with the next generation. Such changes within the community were at times difficult to take. Women related this to general health issues, as Sakeena shows:

County hall was looking for an Asian social worker and I applied and got the job. I worked there for three months in the family and maternity unit so that was another experience, about how teenage pregnancy was in the Asian community. Our people think this doesn't happen, it's such an eye opener . . . shocking because girls are pregnant and not a single family member knows, it's a hidden pregnancy. . . . Now communities are accepting that Hindu girls are wanting to marry Muslim boys, but not this.

Women within the study socialized with other women across religions and this often affected and increased their use of different types of Asian non-Western and at times Western remedies. This socialization across different religions also related to their identification with a much broader sense of an Asian community. Sometimes respondents seemed to see themselves as part of this community and the community influenced their health choices. Women within the research, however, did distinguish between different generations, associating rigid notions of community with their parents' and grandparents' generations. They saw these notions as changing over time, and while older generations played a role in influencing their health choices, within this study, women of the same generation were more influential. This reinforces Goldberg's (1993) argument that we need to move away from approaches that lump ethnic groups together as homogenous entities. Women within the study discussed not only socializing across religion, but also the influence of White communities on their health choices.

Hahlo (1998), in his study on Gujaratis in Bolton, looks at the low number of friendships formed between Gujaratis and White people. He argues that what must not be overlooked are the class differences between those in power and those who labor under them. Women within this study talked primarily about socializing with other Asian women of the same and/or different religions. However, they did also socialize with women from White communities, although, as in Hahlo's study, socialization was relatively low, as Samina demonstrates:

Yes, some of my friends are White, I mean I have Asian friends as well.

The women did talk about White friends at times influencing their health choices. Friends often told the respondents about various remedies to use, including folk, alternative, and biomedical, as Samina points out in talking about the influence of one of her White friends:

My friend Jane is White, yeah she sometimes gives me all kinds of health advice.

These friendships and influences often changed as respondents progressed through the life course. As Shahnaz's account shows, many women within the study felt that they socialized with White women more at school and at work; once they were married, particularly if a woman had given up work, this socialization decreased. After marriage, women within the study socialized more within an Asian community context:

> I did use to feel more part of that [Western culture]. But now because I'm not mixing so much, with Western culture. I don't feel as if I am part of that any more because it doesn't come into my life as much at the moment. [Do you mix mostly within the Muslim community in Leicester now?] Well I don't even feel as if I'm mixing among the Muslim community, just within the family.

Consequently, this decrease of contact impacted on White women's influence on the respondent's health choices. At the time of this research the women's White female friends seemed less influential on the women's health choices than other Asian women or those from the same group. In his study, Hahlo (1998) also distinguishes between degrees of friendship. A relationship based on acquaintanceship carries fewer demands than those imposed by close friendship. Within this study it appeared that while women might have White friends, these were not close friends. Their friendship also decreased over time, which in turn seemed to lessen their influence on health choices. This again emphasizes the need to recognize the complexity of positions held by the women in the study and the impact of such complexity on their health choices. As argued in previous chapters, influences on women's health choices shift over time, as do the choices themselves. Concurring with findings of recent studies on ethnicity and identity (Parker 1995; Woollett, Marshall, Nicolson, and Dosanjh-Matwala 1994), respondents within this study were not caught in a process of increasing "assimilation." Rather, their position as British Asians enabled them to move in and out of differing positions, creating new spaces. In this sense, the respondents' accounts highlight the benefits of the framework of syncrecy, which recognizes tensions between categories and captures the processual nature of health choices.

Jeffers, Hoggett, and Harrison (1996), as noted previously, identify two types of community: that based on people sharing beliefs and values and that configured in spatial terms. Within this book the former has so far been explored through the accounts of the women researched. I now want to move on to begin to explore community influence in more spatial terms (space is explored more thoroughly in Chapter 5). In talking about health choices, women within the study made reference to neighbors' influence and the importance of geographical context. Here respondents drew on community knowledge from those living close by. Neighbors were sometimes, although not exclusively, part of the same religious community. Neighbors seemed to offer a plethora of advice, and respondents seemed to offer them advice in return. Rambha discusses her husband, who had an abscess on his back and consequently suffered a lot of back pain. His doctor recommended when he felt the pain that he lie on a plank of wood. This apparently did the trick and so he passed this information on to a neighbor:

> Yeah, any time he feels the pain now I've got that wood there and he can just lie on it. I mean my neighbor said that he's been given this medicine for his back, my husband says to him if you want my advice you'll get a plank of wood and lie on it, so he did and he feels much better!

For the women within the study, while neighbors may not always be influential on health choices and may be more of a peripheral part of the lay referral network, an absence of such was often felt itself to lead to ill-health, as Sita demonstrates:

> Women suffer from depression because they feel lonely and isolated without close neighbors. . . . You know

when you're cooking and making chapati and accidentally you burn one and you feel upset for a while, but then talking to your neighbors you'll say, "Ohhh I burned my chapatis," see then it's out of your system. Well there are times I've noticed no matter how big the problems you have, if you can express it to others, it's on your mind less.

Neighborly influence also tended to change over time as community groups moved in and out of different areas, as Sakeena shows:

Yes, what has happened is because there is a mosque here so even other people like the Sikh community they all sell, moving from here and it is a highly Muslim dominated area now. Wherever the mosque is near, I know that Muslim people find it very handy because their children are young and they are having to send them there every day.

In her study on working-class communities in the East End of London, Cornwell (1984) found that the importance of community waxed and waned according to the type of interview account. She makes a distinction within her research between public and private interview accounts. Public are those initial statements given within the interview process. Initially people talk less about personal information and talk more generally about health. Private accounts are those given once an interview rapport has been developed; people then talk more freely and personally. In public accounts people emphasized community characteristics of friendliness and concern for others. Their private accounts, however, highlighted the overriding importance of looking after oneself and underlined the diversity of community. Her argument is relevant for women's accounts here (although they cannot be split so crudely into public and private accounts). At times community seemed important within the women's accounts, and at other times this was not so. Within the study, women's accounts highlighted the diversity in extent and type of community influence on their health choices.

In an empirical sense, the term "community" cannot be used holistically. As the accounts of the women show, it incorporates and broadens their family networks and involves a multiplicity of layers, including religion, the broader Asian community, socializing across communities, and spatial and other community influence. These all influence respondents' use of particular remedies in differing times and contexts, and to differing extents. Taken as a whole, they influence respondents' syncretic use of remedies. Community influence highlights the importance of women's position as British Asians. Through this position of being raised in Britain but being part of a broader Asian diasporic network, women are able to move within and between the layers of community, with generation intersecting with community. This in turn influences the respondents' use of syncretic remedies. As argued within this section of the chapter, respondents' relationships to community emphasize the need for an approach that is dynamic and processual, one that moves beyond "between two cultures" approaches. Through their position as British Asians, respondents felt that they actively engaged with differing layers of community, reinscribing them through their syncretic health choices.

Religion and community influence women's syncretic use of remedies, and by process they also reflect the multiple layers of women's identities. It is in this final section of the chapter that the connections between identity, health, and syncrecy will be explored.

IDENTITY AND HEALTH

As argued earlier, in researching people's attitudes toward health we not only get their accounts on health but also information and general claims about their overall identity. As Radley and Billig (1996) argue, people do not merely "have" ideas about their health. They also construct their state of health as part of their ongoing identities in relation to others, as something vital to the conduct of everyday life. Health and illness are a significant part of people's identities, and the onset of illness often involves a renegotiation of those identities (Mathieson and Stam 1995). Accounts given of health and illness are therefore more than a disclosing of an internal attitude. In offering views, people are also making claims about themselves as worthy individuals, as more or less fit participants in the social world. Within accounts, personal and social conditions of identity formation continuously interconnect. "Autobiographical reflections constantly draw on wider social developments, which are framed and understood in terms of personal and familial narratives. Cultural identities are constructed through the alignment of personal and collective memories and stories" (Parker 1995, 242).

Earlier in this book the theoretical framework of syncrecy was developed, drawing on approaches used within the study of ethnicity and identity. As Solomos (1988) demonstrates, in much of the literature children of postwar migrants were seen as problems, stranded between two cultures, in conflict with their parents and facing the difficulties of two incommensurable value systems. Within studies on identity, dissatisfaction with "between two cultures" approaches and identity conflicts has led to a move away from static and rigid attributions of identity to a conception of identity less as a fixed entity, a readily measurable attribute, or a construal, and more as a process, an ongoing construction (Griffin 1989).

There is a general reconception of identity through the analysis of diasporic cultures. In talking about the positioning of second-generation Asians within Britain, Kelleher (1996), suggests that rather than being situated between two cultures, this generational group draws on both parent and Western cultures in different ways and in differing contexts. As argued throughout this and other chapters, the concept of syncrecy is used in this context to explore and denote crossovers and tensions between categories of difference, both British–Asian and Western–non-Western (Parker 1995). With a focus on both crossover and tension between categories, the concept of syncrecy, rather than fostering a "between two cultures" approach, is a transformative concept allowing for fluidity and change.

Within this study, as women were talking about syncretic health choices they also talked about their syncretic identities. Women within the study often identified themselves as both British and Asian at the same time, as Surinder and Gurinder show:

> I am British but then I'm Asian at the same time but I wouldn't say I'm totally Westernized, not like some women my age. I know some of them are English in the way they dress.

> I think I class myself as Asian. I'd say I'm Asian because that's the upbringing I've had and the culture I've had but I've had Western influence as well. I've had the best of both worlds. Yes, I'm British Asian, I wouldn't say that I was Asian wouldn't say I'm British. I'm British Asian, a mix of both.

This identification as British Asian has multiple layers. While women within the study sometimes liked to identify as British Asian, at other times they talked in much more religious terms, for instance, identifying more as British Muslims with an Asian background, as Samina stresses:

> Yeah, that's right and I'm a Muslim, yeah I'd like to be a strong Muslim you know and do what we're supposed to do but because we've been born here and brought up here and we've socialized in a way with children of different religions and we've seen everything and so want to be a part of it 'cause that's where we've been from the beginning.

This layering of identity again highlights the need, as Solomos (1988) argues, to move away from approaches that try and fix the identity of children of postwar migrants, allocating them "between two cultures." As the accounts of the women researched here suggest, identity is much more processual and syncretic.

Hahlo (1998), in his study on ethnicity, community, and politics among Gujaratis in Bolton, highlights this multiple layering of identity. He argues that in relation to members of other ethnic groups or White communities, Gujaratis often describe themselves as Gujaratis. However, when differentiating themselves and other Gujaratis they distinguish between belonging to a community such as a caste community and others belonging to other caste communities. Women within this study differentiated themselves in similar ways, although this was not necessarily based in spatial terms, as with Hahlo's respondents. Rather, women moved in and out of categories of religion to broader categories of Asian identification. Again, this was reflected in health choice, as demonstrated earlier through religion and the multiple layers of community.

In Chapter 3 I looked at the clash in health choices between women within the study who identified as British Asian and husbands who were from India. This clash often led to health problems for the women. This can be translated into general conflicts in identity between women born in the United Kingdom and husbands from India, as Samina demonstrates:

> Yeah, I'd say I was British Muslim, that's what I'd like to say 'cos that's the way that I can identify myself because that's what it is you know like. I'll say to my husband when we're having a row or something you know or if we're talking I say, "Shut up, I'm British you know," and he will say, "Look at you you're not exactly English are you." My husband he's from back home [India] and we do have a lot of differences because of that. You know 'cos that's when I realize that there is a lot of difference between people from back home, no matter how long they've lived here they still go back to India.

As argued earlier, respondents' health choices change over time as they progress throughout the life course. This is re-

flected in the identity of the respondents, and their identification as British Asians changing as they get married and
have children. Woollett et al. (1994), in their study on gender, ethnicity, and identity among South Asian women in
London, focus on changes in ethnic identity over time as
women marry and have children. They argue that over time
women adopt a lifestyle of the dominant culture, but this is
not just about increased familiarity with culture. Changes
are also related to the women's own position within the life
course, changing in particular on becoming a mother. Within
the women's accounts, women identified changes in their
identity over the life course. This involved a pull to and away
from Westernization, emphasizing a syncretic tension, a position more fluid and complex than one couched between
two cultures. Some women often identified their identity as
changing over time as they progressed from young working
women through to marriage and motherhood (see Chapter
3). Often this involved moving through different states of
influence, as Shahnaz shows:

> I think as I've got older and especially since I've stopped
> work and I've got kids and everything. At this moment
> in time I see myself more as a Muslim person with an
> Indian background. Whereas whilst I was still working
> and before I was married and everything I saw myself
> as British Indian you know. I tended to feel more Brit-
> ish. I feel "now" more [pause] my lifestyle's changed
> especially since I've finished work I'm usually at home.
> I'm very restricted in my social circle. It tends to nar-
> row the field a lot and it does obviously alter your out-
> look on how you see yourself and how people see you.

In talking about their health choices, women within the
study made claims about their identity. In general, most
women identified as British Asian; at times this varied in
specificity, with women often identifying themselves by religion. These differing categories can come into conflict, particularly for women married to men born in India, East Africa,

and so on. These categories also transform themselves as women progress throughout the life course.

In moving through time, different layers of respondents' identities become more central to them at certain times, and this translates down to their health choices. For instance, religion, as shown in the previous section, is sometimes a particularly significant part of the identities of the women within the study. Sometimes being Muslim or Sikh overrode other aspects of women's identity. This was reflected in respondents' health choices and became a central influence on their use of different types of remedies. As already argued, in some women's accounts, at particular times such as during pregnancy and childbirth, religion seemed very important in influencing their health choices. The consumption of "hot" and "cold" foods at certain points of the pregnancy seemed to be particularly important for Muslim women in the research. The Hindu and Sikh women within the study were less focused on diet in pregnancy and did not talk about food in terms of "hot" and "cold" properties. At other times differing factors appeared more prevalent parts of the respondents' identities than religion. For example, in looking at community influence, sometimes women identified with a much broader category of Asian and this was reflected in women's health choices (this will be discussed further in the conclusion). On occasion women within the study drew heavily on advice from Asian women of other religious communities. This enabled women to use non-Western remedies not necessarily associated with religion.

Women within the study moved through these different states of identity and differing influences on their health choices. These influences are in dialogue with one another. They also conflict and contradict one another as differing contextual influences fight for recognition. Differing contextual circumstances influence syncretic use of remedies in differing contexts, determined historically, locally, and personally. This point is explored more fully in the conclusion to this book. These parts of the respondents identities and influences on health choices are not seen as fixed but as continually shifting and being reconfigured in the light of change, depending on what they were talking about, who they were talking to, and their temporal location. It is important to recognize that any one part of the respondents' identities, such as class or religion, may be more important at any one time, and that these interrelate across the women's accounts, fostering syncretic identities and health choices.

CONCLUSION

Religion and community can thus be seen as significant influences on the health choices made by the women in this research. Such influence, however, is far from homogeneous. Rather, influence varies according to religion and community type and also shifts across time. Such an analysis highlights a degree of cohesiveness here among women of the same religion. However, this does not necessarily mean that women of the same religion adhere to the same practices, or that non-Western remedies associated with particular religions are necessarily homogeneous. It must also be recognized, as Porter and Hinnells (1999) point out, that religions are far from internally cohesive.

The idea of community is also far from homogeneous. The women's accounts can be seen to reinforce the idea that the concept of community is fluid and layered. As Alexander (1996) and others have argued, people cannot be fixed into specific community types. Community rather is fluid, layered, and context specific. In this context, such a layering of community emphasizes the shifting influence of generation, gender, and ethnicity on health choices. When we look at community, sometimes women of similar ages but of different religious or ethnic groups are more influential, emphasizing the primacy of generation. At other times older women of the same ethnic and religious group are most influential, emphasizing the importance of ethnic group affiliation. In all cases, both in terms of friendship and community, women mostly talked about the influence of other women on health choices. This highlights the gendered nature of both community and friendship.

Identity has become a growth area within sociology. Key debates on identity have focused on the issue of whether identity is a completely fixed entity or whether it is fluid and changing over time (Bradley 1996). Within the substantive areas of ethnicity and health, debates on identity have been taken up in particular ways. On the one hand, studies on ethnicity have focused on the complex nature of identity for second- and third-generation ethnic groups. On the other hand, within health studies links have been made between people's descriptions of their health and their sense of self. The women's accounts within this study point to an integration of the two. The women's sense of identity, of being British Asians, affects their use of syncretic remedies. This confirms the idea that identity is fluid.

In demonstrating the significance of religion and community on health choices and the reflections of identity in health accounts, the importance of spatial context on health choices has begun to be explored. Within the women's accounts, the women's location in Leicester and their connections with the Asian diaspora in India and other contexts is very influential on health choices. It is to these I will now turn.

Chapter 5

Location, Space, and Globalization

In the previous chapter I explored the influence of religion and community on women's health choices. I argued that both influenced women's syncretic use of remedies at different times and in different contexts, and situated this use within the wider context of identity. Within the section on community I also referred to the influence of space and location on women's health choices. This chapter explores the influence of space in more detail. Space, geographical location, and the reciprocal nature of globalization are all significant variables of influence for the women within this study. What became apparent within women's accounts is the importance of their location in Leicester and their connections and resources within India. Women identified their location in Leicester as giving them access to a variety of health remedies. Women's connections with India also geographically extend their access to a plurality of medicines. These connections are strengthened by processes inherent within globalization, fostering the transcultural flow of syncretic health goods and enabling the respondents' syncretic use of remedies within India. Syncrecy is then opened up in local and global contexts.

Existing literature on space and geographies of health has come from two very broad approaches. The first takes a top-down approach and focuses on the globalization of health systems (B. Turner 1987). This focus maps the globalization of health systems in political terms, focusing on free-enterprise systems, welfare forms, and transitional and socialist types, and maps these systems in different geographical contexts. In this approach medicine in the modern period is mapped along the world economic system, which has become the common basis for a number of institutional responses to illness and mortality. Taking a slightly different angle, other top-ended approaches have focused on geographical inequalities in health and health care. Such studies in geographical inequalities have often been based on epidemiological research. These studies have often focused on inequality along gender, race, and class lines as well as on divides in health between Northern and Southern countries (Doyal 1995).

The second approach takes the opposite focus, which is more anthropological and historical and focuses on geographically mapping plural medicine. It takes a historically comparative approach to the issue of plural medicine in different countries. The approach includes historical explorations of the existence of plural medicine in various geographical locations; for instance, the coexistence of Unani Tibb, Ayurveda, Sidha, and Western medicine in India and their spread to other parts of the globe through migrants (particularly to the Arab world). The spread of these systems is diverse. As Meade, Horin, and Gesler (1988) argue, some medical systems tend to be spatially static, while others have diffused over wide areas. In either case, the result is that various systems overlap in the same space and that most people have a choice of medical systems.

This focus on plural medicine also fits in with current debates on the growth of alternative medicine in the West and the reemergence of plural medicine in so-called Western contexts. As West (1992) argues, alternative medicine is witnessing an increase on a global level, particularly in Western countries. Worsley (1997) argues that today Western medicine has become the single most influential kind of medicine globally. It has achieved a degree of cultural hegemony that enables powerful states and corporations to extend their global reach and influence. At the same time, traditional kinds of medicine not only continue to exist but have spread outside the areas of origin, and new ones are constantly spreading and developing. In the medical sphere, then, culture and structure are by no means congruent with the nation–state. These types of approaches are further diffused through qualitative studies, referred to in Chapter 1, that follow migrant and minority health choices and experiences of health and health care and plural medicine in Western contexts.

Both of these approaches touch on the findings relating to space and health in this study, particularly the latter. The latter approach highlights the ways in which medical systems become diffused over geographical areas, both past and present. This helps us to explore respondents' potential access to plural medicine in Leicester and elsewhere through their membership in a particularly mobile diasporic group with associated medical systems. These approaches, however, do not really enable us to explore how these connections between diasporic groups and contexts are so readily possible for the respondents within this study. In order to explore this more thoroughly, I draw on a third body of literature that focuses more heavily on wider debates on globalization. One cannot talk about respondents' use of health care in India and the transcultural flow of health products without referring to these debates. Massey (1994) has argued that we are now living through a period of intense spatial upheaval, an era of new and powerful globalization, of instantaneous worldwide communications, of the breakup of what was once local coherence, of a new phase of time and space compression. It is argued that a new global space of electronic information and power relations is emerging.

More generally, it is argued that culture is being globalized through the emergence of global products, the popularity of world music, and so on. The link between culture and place, it is argued, is being ruptured. Each geographical "place" in the world is being realigned in relation to the new global realities. Places within the wider whole are being reassigned, their boundaries dissolved, and they are increasingly crossed by everything from investment flow, to cultural influences, to satellite networks. This is reflected in women's accounts through their frequent travel within the United Kingdom and to India for health reasons. It is also reflected in the transcultural movements of health goods. There appear to be no barriers to respondents' access to plural health care in plural contexts, enabling them to carry out syncretic practices in a plurality of locations.

However, what is apparent in the accounts of the women researched is that at the same time as they move to the global, there is also a return to the local and place-bound traditions. Friedman (1994) argues that when looking at global process one cannot just talk about a move to globalization in terms of cultural decentralization. He argues that what is important to recognize is the interplay between the world market and cultural identity, between local and global processes, between consumption and cultural strategies. The local and, in particular, women's location in Leicester becomes particularly important within this study in influencing respondents' syncretic use of remedies. As Hall (1992b) argues, we must not simply condemn globalization as cultural homogenization. He identifies the oppositional nature of postmodernity, the return to the local as a response to the seeming homogenization and globalization of culture. In following Hall (1992b), it is important to recognize the interplay of these two, both local and global, within women's accounts and to see not one or the other as in some sense purer.

This chapter continues many themes prevalent throughout the book, but situates these within a bigger picture. Within this chapter I will explore the influence of the respondents' location in Leicester on their syncretic use of remedies. The women within the study feel that their location in Leicester gives them access to a variety of types of medicine that they then draw on syncretically. The respondents' employment of such products will again be explored within the context of their position as British Asians, as women socialized within the West who are also part of a wider, globally dispersed ethnic group. Again, the dynamism of this position is emphasized against static between two cultures' approaches. This section will also explore the respondents' use of other non-Western remedies, particularly in the context of global increases in alternative medicine in general. Second, I will explore the way in which women within the study take and bring back a plurality of health goods to and from India. This transcultural flow of goods highlights the significance of the South Asian diasporic network, enabling women the potential to draw on syncretic types of medicine in a multiplicity of locations. This potential to draw on these medical remedies in different locations is made easier through the globalization process. In its emphasis on the deconstruction of borders and boundaries, globalization makes possible the movement of goods between the local and the global. Drawing on arguments made in the previous chapter, such processes of globalization open up the possibility for connections between the diaspora in differing contexts to become real; that is, based on face-to-face interaction. These connections, once only imagined, become real when respondents visit India and other Asian diasporic contexts.

Within the last section of the chapter I will explore the respondents' syncretic use of health products and services within India. Again, this emphasizes the respondents' connections through diasporic networks and the fostering of such links through globalization. Women within the study are able to connect regularly with members of the South Asian diaspora in other locations. This has opened up access to health products and services for women within the study. However, this use of health products and services among the respondents is not straightforwardly unanimous. I will also explore the influence of respondents' locational backgrounds (i.e., respondents with an Indian background, those with an East

African background) on their use of syncretic remedies in India, with East African women within the study being less likely to draw on syncretic remedies in either India or East Africa.

LOCALIZING THE GLOBAL:
LEICESTER IN A NATIONAL CONTEXT

As argued in the introduction, according to 1991 census data (Leicester City Council 1991b) Leicester ranks fifth in terms of absolute numbers of all ethnic minorities, second for all Asian groupings, first for its population of Indian origin, but only thirty-fifth for those who classified themselves as Black. However, outside the London area it is the local authority with the highest percentage of all ethnic minorities. According to the same census data, 23.7 percent of the population of the district of Leicester are of Asian origin. This is compared with 71.5 percent White, 2.4 percent Black, and 2.4 percent ethnic other (Leicester City Council 1991b). While Leicester's Asian population includes Ugandan, Kenyan, Tanzanian, Punjabi, Pakistani, and Bangladeshi, the population is heavily weighted toward East African Asians and Gujarati people, both Muslim and Hindu. As argued in Chapter 3, several women within the study had moved from other parts of England to Leicester to marry. Such women came mostly from Blackburn, Birmingham, and London. The women from Blackburn were all Muslim, those from Birmingham were Sikh, and those from London were Sikh, Muslim, and Hindu. The majority of women who had been born in Leicester were Hindu. Within the study there were six women with an East African background, twenty-two with an Indian background (two of whom had migrated to the United Kingdom via other parts of Europe), one with a Pakistani background, and one with a background in the Caribbean. Fourteen women (those not British born) had migrated to Britain from either East Africa, India, or Pakistan, with one respondent from Trinidad. Women in the study from countries other than Britain had quite frequently moved through several places in Britain before marrying and settling in Leicester.

Jeffers, Hoggett, and Harrison (1996) argue that Leicester is a city where boundary-crossing interactions between various minority and White populations are significant. According to the women's accounts from this study, it also has a close-knit traditional Asian community when compared to other areas, such as Blackburn and London, which have smaller and more scattered populations. Because of the significant amount of people moving to Leicester to marry, these regional differences become mixed. Respondents tie this in with the large South Asian population and its concentration in particular areas of Leicester. As Gurinder suggests,

> Yeah, there's a lot of Asians here like they've kept their traditional values whereas if you're scattered around you've got no option but to mix in and let go with a lot of your culture, so I think that does make it difficult but I mean in London they have their towns that are just like Leicester, you know with lots of Asians. But where we lived in London, it was just mixed.

Many women within the study talked about how racially mixed Leicester is and how this impacts on choice and use of (Western) health care. On discussing the respondents' preference for either a White or Asian doctor, some women within the study preferred to have a White doctor. However, because Leicester has a large Asian population and because Asian communities were housed in the same locations, Asian doctors were often the only option. As Samina, a Muslim woman originating from Blackburn and living in Leicester, commented,

> No actually I prefer a White English doctor yeah, but here, since I've moved to Leicester in the last six years I think I've seen more of the Asian community, well I think that 80 percent of the population is Asian, that's what I've noticed. I mean Blackburn's a little town there,

but there's a lot of Asian people there but at school you
see White children. In the doctor's surgeries you see
White people, whereas here, if I do see a White person I
think, yeah, hello.

Such an emphasis on Leicester's significant South Asian
population as compared to other places in Britain is reflected
in the census data. If we look at the total Asian population in
Birmingham, it stands at 13.5 percent; the population in
Bradford is 13.3 percent. Both areas are known to have large
South Asian populations. In terms of total Asian population,
Leicester stands second only to Tower Hamlets, with an Asian
population of 24.7 percent (Leicester City Council 1991b).
Respondents also identified this large Asian population in
Leicester as affecting their health choices.

"Don't Forget the Tiger Balm": Syncrecy in Leicester

Women within the study felt that their location within
Leicester gave them access to a plurality of health remedies,
both in terms of products and services. This enabled them to
draw on syncretic health remedies. Within the study, however, a distinction was made in terms of use of services and
products, with respondents drawing more heavily on products. In terms of Asian medical services, Leicester has one
Ayurvedic clinic. There are also a number of Hakims who
practice the Muslim medical system Unani, a faculty of Tibb
Eastern medicine. While being aware that Vaida and Hakim
clinics existed in Leicester, views on the availability and use
of the services and satisfaction with them were mixed.
Hakims were quite widely talked about and many women
knew of clinics and practitioners. Sakeena talked about her
knowledge of alternative practitioners:

I know one Hakim in Leicester, up on Evington road. I
also know an acupuncturist, our doctor's surgery is now
including acupuncture.

Most of the women within the study were quite cynical about them though and saw Hakims and Vaidas as unsatisfactory and too expensive. Sita's account was not uncommon among respondents:

> There was this guy, this Vaida, he charges you £25 per session and after four sessions he will tell you if you are going to be fully cured or not. I mean he's got a £100 out of me and after that he says you're not going to be cured, why should I, you know, throw my money away in the bin as well as my confidence?

Many women within the study were worried about coming into contact with someone who was not properly qualified. This applied to both Ayurvedic clinics and Hakims. As Sita remarked,

> Yes, now that holds me back, what if I come into contact with someone who isn't fully qualified? People practice and they say they are qualified but I don't know, somehow I'm reluctant to use it.

This line of argument is supported by Karseras and Hopkins (1987), who suggest that while healers on the subcontinent must be qualified, this is not so in Britain. Anyone can call themselves a Vaida or a Hakim, with the obvious danger that patients suffering from a serious but potentially treatable condition could be consulting an untrained person with little experience. Women within the study were less likely to hold these types of views about Western medical practitioners in Leicester.

Within the study, access to Asian products appeared to be far more important than use of Asian medical services. Women were much more likely to use Asian products than they were to actually visit official Asian medical healers. In talking about the availability of products in Leicester, Samina, a Muslim originally from Blackburn, argued,

> In Leicester I've seen it [laughs], you can get everything in Leicester. Where I come from, in Blackburn, we al-

ways get them sent down from India. Tiger balm, don't
forget the Tiger Balm!

This was a commonly held view, particularly when women
within the study talked about balms for general health. As
discussed in previous chapters, women within the study also
talked about the availability of "Asian" herbs within Leicester for general health. As Kishwar shows,

> Highfields or Melton Road, there are lots of like herb
> shops, selling Asian herbs you know to use for general
> health, Jaipur mill etc. cash and carrys and places like
> that, its easy to get that stuff in Leicester.

Sakeena related this issue of significant availability of health
products in Leicester to the multicultural nature of the city:

> I think the reason is, it is easier to get here because it's
> very multicultural in Leicester and Leicester is not a
> very big city. I suppose if you don't find one thing in
> Evington area about a ten-minute drive and you can, or
> Highfields you can find it. Say you were living in Lon-
> don and you live in the east, you have to go up west
> and get your products and that takes ages.

Women within the study appeared very proud of their
knowledge of these products and even of Asian health care
within Leicester. I would argue this gives us our first example
of what Clifford (1997) calls "diaspora discourse," which
blends together notions of both host and homeland, connect-
ing members of the South Asian diaspora in a number of
locations and aiding access to a plurality of products and
services. Health goods flow between members of the South
Asian diaspora in different locations, from Leicester through
other national and international contexts.

Many respondents talked about the use of health products
or health care that were neither Western nor South Asian.
Women within the study also went to visit alternative practi-

tioners such as those practicing acupuncture; this was mostly for general illness, such as hay fever, and bodily aches and pains. Kishwar talked about her husband's use of other alternatives:

> I have taken my husband to a Chinese herbalist just off Evington Road. It was to do with his hay fever.

Women within the study went to other cities in order to get certain treatments or to visit particular healers. Respondents found out about alternative practitioners and clinics in other contexts through friends' recommendations. They often sought out healers in other places when they had exhausted health care resources within Leicester. Kishwar discusses going to visit other healers in other places:

> Someone at lunch mentioned that there is a herbalist in Manchester who is from Saudi Arabia and I've said yes to going to see him.

Indian health care services and, more important, health care products are reasonably widely available in Leicester. Other types, such as traditional Chinese medicine, though available, are less easy to find in Leicester. Cant and Sharma (1999) argue that many British studies have shown that there are regional differences in the use of alternative health care. The north of England has much lower levels of consultation (MORI 1989). This may, however, reflect the greater number of practitioners and training schools in the south (Thomas 1989). Southern bias regarding some alternative therapies such as reflexology, chiropractors, and homeopaths perhaps affects respondents' use of some therapies (Cant and Sharma 1999). Respondents' position as British Asiana, as members of an ethnic group in a location with a significant South Asian population with broader diasporic connections, gives them access to Asian medicine. A small Chinese population in Leicester (22% Indian compared to 0.3% Chinese; Leicester City Council 1991b) may also limit the availability and use of traditional Chinese medicine by the respondents.

Respondents' use of a broad range of non-Western products is related to their dissatisfaction with Western health care services within Leicester, as Lata, a Hindu respondent, suggests:

> Well, we weren't happy about the care we were getting with the GP or at the Royal [Leicester Royal Infirmary] so we decided to try some alternatives, it made sense to.

This reflects the broader picture of an overall growth within Britain in the use of alternative health care. It fits in with general arguments (made throughout the book) about dissatisfaction with approaches in Western health care. As Worsley (1997) argues, many people in Britain, after consulting their GP, feel dissatisfied and experiment with non-Western medicine. Women in the study were on the whole quite keen to use alternatives, although none expressed a desire to completely replace Western remedies with alternative practices. As Gurinder explained, women also linked increased use of alternative health care with more general shifts in the National Health Service (NHS) and Western society in general:

> I think it is age but it is also with the way society is. I mean it is not always the answer and the doctors don't always diagnose you the right way. I think it is the way the NHS is going.

It is important to recognize power dynamics within this global spread of non-Western medicine. It must also be located within the argument of the wider issue of the power of global marketing and health (Morley and Robins 1995). The marketing of cultural products through the electronic mediascape is important.This indicates a celebration of ethnic difference in a very postmodern sense, making difference not only acceptable but also fashionable.

Despite the skepticism of respondents toward Western health care in Leicester, they did tend to use non-Western medicine syncretically with Western medicine at different times and for different reasons. As Jameela shows,

Well you know it's good because I can get my balms
and stuff in Leicester, like tiger balm and that. But I do
go to my doctor and get stuff from the chemist, you know,
like paracetemol.

As argued throughout the book, respondents identified
their position as British Asians as giving them access to a
range of cultural resources not readily available to other populations in Leicester. This relates to their membership within
a wider diasporic network. As British Asians, women in the
study occupy a unique position that is more dynamic than
one caught between two cultures. Respondents have access
to both Western and non-Western medicine through Western socialization and as part of an ethnic minority group that
is geographically dispersed. Because of the ability of diasporas to connect multiple communities, women within the
study were able to access a whole range of products and services within Leicester. In particular, respondents' location
in Leicester and their position as British Asian women enabled them to draw on syncretic remedies, drawing on both
Western and Asian medicine. While other alternative remedies were not quite as available within Leicester, women
within the study still drew on them when feasible. This also
highlights, at a general level, the increase in alternative medicines. Within the next section I will look at how the use of
these syncretic products extends from along local and national lines to global contexts, focusing on the transcultural
flow of goods and capital.

FROM HERE TO INDIA (AND BACK): THE
TRANSCULTURAL FLOW OF HEALTH PRODUCTS

Much of the literature on globalization (Clifford 1997) looks
at how separate places become effectively a single community through the continuous circulation of people, money,
goods, and information. This culturally homogenizing type
of argument has been heavily criticized; as Grewal and Kaplan
(1994) argue, such reference to transcultural flows of goods

should be seen instead as scattered hegemonies that are the effects of mobile capital as well as the multiple subjectivities that replace the unitary European subject. As other authors have pointed out, the movements of any forms of capital in a global era should not be seen as one-way flows. Relating to health, Worsley (1997) argues that today the flow of people and ideas across the globe is so great that cultural exchanges overcome political barriers. He argues that though Western remedies may diffuse particularly rapidly, the traffic is not all one way. Within the context of diasporas, globalization with its deconstruction of borders and boundaries makes it possible for products and people to traverse diasporic networks particularly efficiently. This current phase of globalization enables the possibility of connections between Asian diasporas in the United Kingdom, Asians in Asia, and diasporas in other locations to become "real" at certain times; that is, based on face-to-face contact. These connections for first-generation migrants during the 1960s and 1970s were mostly only "imagined."

This is reflected in respondents' accounts when they talk about how they buy health products, both Western and Asian, from other contexts and bring them back to the United Kingdom, and also how they take certain things to other countries. Women within the study move syncretic products reciprocally between India and Britain. This occurs when respondents are on holiday or visiting family. Such exchanges mostly take place between Britain and India. I argue that rather than seeing this as evidence of either cultural renaissance or homogenization, it relates rather to the push and pull of both local and global forces, which form part of the process of globalization as national boundaries are opened. Women within the study go over to India to buy non-Western and Western health products, which are then circulated within the local context. At the same time the reciprocity of the local–global process is emphasized through taking goods to India and dispersing them within family networks there. As Sita explained,

I take multivitamin tablets, my family in India really like us to take them if anybody's going over [to India].

Women within the study took health products from the United Kingdom to family in India and various other places because family members saw them as better than products available there. These were mostly things like vitamin tablets and painkillers. Women within the study also talked about certain products they went to India to buy. In discussions on cultural pluralism, India is often cited as a premier example (Meade, Horin, and Gesler 1988). It has many variations in language, religion, and social status and other cultural traits. Such pluralism is also reflected within health care in India, with Ayurveda, Sidha, and Unani being prevalent from the fifteenth and sixteenth centuries, followed by the subsequent implementation of biomedicine (Meade, Horin, and Gesler 1988). Women within the study drew on such plural health systems in India syncretically. Respondents' need to draw on these resources in India depended on their location in the United Kingdom. Women in Leicester, as already demonstrated, could access most South Asian balms from Leicester. Kishwar and many other women within the study went to India to buy non-Western goods already available in Leicester, mostly because they were cheaper in India as there you do not pay VAT:

Oh yeah, I always stock up on everything when I go over there [India]. I mean it's cheaper there. You probably pay a few Rupees over there and £3 for the same thing here. My stock comes mostly from there, but if I was desperate I know that I could still buy things from here if it was a problem.

Respondents had to go to India to obtain some Asian balms. There were also other non-Western skin products that women within the study bought in India that are unavailable in Britain. As Gurinder, a Sikh, argued,

My dad has psoriasis and he's had medicine from India for that. There's this special tablet that I think is specifically for people with eczema and psoriasis. It worked on him; it is like a little herbal remedy you get from India.

Other goods that respondents went to India to buy specifically were herbal tablets for diabetes. Some women also went to India for specific Western health products, because certain things are available there that are not in Britain. Ramila, a Hindu, talked about going to India for diet pills:

Next time I go [to India] I want to get a diet pill that makes you lose weight, that you can't get here. You can get that there. You know amphetamine, what you used to be able to get here but are banned now.

Again, within the research the women's position as British Asians affected their access to a plurality of health resources. This was most notable in two different ways: British Asian women appear to have greater access to Asian medical products and services because they are part of an ethnic group with greater access to products and services through the South Asian diasporic network. The women's status as part of a mobile group with a significantly globally dispersed network also heightens access to both Western and non-Western products in other contexts. This again illuminates the respondents' position as dynamic. It enables women within the study to draw on syncretic remedies within contexts other than the United Kingdom. These types of cultural exchanges on a global level have been demonstrated in other research on diasporic communities, though not relating to exchanges in health products. Parker (1995) argues in his research on British Chinese that their connections to places of origin are made through material exchanges. Cultural commodities from Hong Kong are exported within days to distribution companies in France, North America, and London.

Some women within the study felt quite cautious about either sending things to India or bringing them from India back to Britain. This is because they were cautious over the content of products bought in India. This could also be related to respondents' caution about breaking the law regarding nonpayment of tax duties and importation of banned goods. Women within the study would sometimes talk about buying and bringing things back only when someone else had already tried it. As Gurinder said,

If I, or my husband, had an illness such as psoriasis and someone told me "Oh there is this medicine from India," I would try it. If I knew someone else that had used it and I knew that it had benefited them then I would try it.

Women within the study also talked about the flow of labor between countries (in this case India and Britain) and the way in which people received work qualifications in different countries. When talking about biomedical doctors in India, many women talked about how they got their medical training in the United Kingdom or America. Musarat said,

But you know, sometimes even the doctors there [India], I'm not saying they're qualified here [United Kingdom] and not there, they get their training over here. Yeah, then they go back. Most people come over here, London or Cambridge.

This often impacted whether women trusted doctors in India.

Within the study, women's position as British Asians, as part of a globally dispersed group, gives them the connections enabling them to draw on a plurality of remedies in other contexts. Globalization, with its emphasis on time–space compression, deconstruction of borders and boundaries, global telecommunications, cheap air travel, and so on, fosters connections between them and diaspora in other contexts and India. It enables the respondents to spatially extend their syncretic use of remedies, making "imagined" connections between diaspora in different times and contexts (and homelands) become "real." Through such positions and processes women within the study were able to draw on syncretic remedies cross-nationally, moving products between India and Britain. It must be recognized here that women within the study make these trips regardless of socioeconomic position. All women within the study had made trips to India at some point.

In the next section I will extend some of the arguments made here to explore the way in which women within the study, through similar processes, use products and services syncretically within India.

Using Syncretic Health Products and Services in India

Many women within the study were open to using Western health care in India, or had used health care there generally if they needed to when visiting. It was also common for respondents to use health facilities in India for specific treatments. Musarat talks about someone going to India from Britain specifically for eye treatments:

When we went over to India we met up with this guy. He had an eye problem and he went over there specifically because of this eye problem and he was a lot better. He had an operation in India and he was a lot better, he lived here [United Kingdom] in Walsall.

Some women within the study even had family doctors in India, in case they needed to use one when they visited family. Respondents often explained this use of health care in India by reference to its cheapness. However, it also appeared that women used it because of marked differences in care between Britain and India, and in some respects treatment seemed better in India. This reflects Worsley's (1997) argument that despite the internationalism of Western medicine, marked cultural differences persist in each country. Women within the study talked about how you could go private in

India and pay a lot less but get good treatments; Gurinder related this to being viewed there as being "from abroad":

> To them 100 or 200 rupees, it is like private so, and getting your best treatment just for a little bit more so I would prefer to. You know that little extra care, particularly if you're from abroad; they do treat you a lot better in India.

Women within the study went to India for various treatments because they felt that they were performed better there, and many talked about how they used health care in India when they felt they were not being treated properly in the United Kingdom. As discussed in Chapter 2, Shahnaz talked about how her sister-in-law's husband died of cancer. He had been misdiagnosed in the United Kingdom so went to India and was treated more promptly, albeit too late to save his life:

> He wasn't actually seen [by a doctor] until the September of 1996, they said there wasn't anything wrong with him. In December he was getting worse. He changed GPs and the new GP realized it was bad and finally got things rolling. The state of his health deteriorated so much that he eventually went to India. Within the first doctor, the first examination he had, they diagnosed him as having cancer.

Shahnaz felt that if her relative had finished his treatment in India he might have survived. Such dissatisfaction with Western health care was located in the women's accounts around more general arguments about poor standards within the National Health Service. Women within the study on the whole complained about waiting lists, inability getting appointments, and poor or wrong diagnoses. While many authors have talked about the poor treatment of minorities and migrants generally within the health service, relating this to racism (Ahmad 1993), women within the study were reluctant to talk about inadequacies as a result of racist practices (see Chapter 2). This may or may not be related to the problematic nature of interviewing across race. Respondents were keener to attribute unhappiness with the health services to a general deterioration in health care.

In this sense, using health care both generally and for specific reasons and in emergencies in India can be seen as a pragmatic alternative for these British Asian women to health care in the United Kingdom. India can be interpreted as a site open only to Indians or diasporic Indians because of connections; it is not open in the same way to White British people. Rather than seeing this move to health care in India as a quest for authenticity, we must analytically reframe such quests amid a widening field of available positions of pragmatism (Bausinger 1990; Narayan 1996). As Shahnaz demonstrates, India opens up possibilities for women as consumers of health products and services that are not as accessible for White Britons and other populations:

> You shouldn't need to go to India to get treated. We [Asians] have got some place to go to but what about White people who are born here. They haven't got another country to go to, you know.

However, women within the study often argued that although they would use biomedicine within India and were glad they had that option if needed, they would nevertheless prefer to use health care in the United Kingdom if they had the choice. As Samina shows, she would ultimately rather be treated in Britain because she was born in Britain:

> I'd rather be treated over here personally. I don't know why, I've just got this thing with them. Because I was born here.

Mostly when respondents talked about using health care in India it was Western health care. However, women within the study did use some non-Western remedies within India, marking an overall syncretic use of remedies there. One woman had used a Hakim while in India, and some women went to practitioners who used herbal remedies and religious and spiritual healers. Sita argued that whether you used non-Western health care in India depended on what kinds of family contacts you had within a wider diasporic context; whether, for instance, you had Ayurvedic practitioners in your family:

> What sort of background they have, like I was saying, my grandfather was very much into Ayurveda but still once he passed away we would rather stick to a normal [Western] doctor over there. In India your GP is like your family member, it's literally like, you know it's called a family doctor.

When possible, women within the study did draw on a variety of remedies in India. Respondents' accounts again highlight the way in which their syncretic use of remedies has a global dimension, substantially transcending local specificity. Kishwar, a Muslim respondent, illustrated this when she talked about using health care for fertility problems in many diverse contexts:

> Due to having problems having children, the doctor diagnosed that there was a problem with him [her husband]. So we had to go to various herbalists from India, people's recommendations and things, and we've also been to like private and medication like BUPA and even like to Harley Street in London.

Women within the study drew on syncretic remedies in contexts beyond national boundaries. Women within the study also drew on remedies from different places syncretically, as Shahnaz shows:

> I mean it doesn't matter whether it's a GP here [in Leicester] or a GP there [India], or a religious or herbal healer here or there. Whatever, you keep them in conjunction and use them at different times.

Such use of health care and products in a variety of contexts can also be related to Giddens's (1991b) formulation about reflexivity and health. He discusses the increase in patient reflexivity, knowledgeability, and choice in relation to health care. He identifies choice in many aspects of life as an obligatory part of posttraditional society. While respondents chose to draw on health care in a number of contexts, many of them were also very wary of using health care (just as they were with health products) in India, either Western or non-Western. This places caution on the extent of respondents' health choices. They were fearful, as they felt doctors and other medical professionals might not be properly qualified there. As Gurinder commented,

If I was there, I wouldn't go, personally, because you are dubious in India because doctors aren't, you know, qualified. You know here because they've got their medical certificates and stuff, but in India I don't know doctors scare me a bit because you hear stories. That patients go to the doctor's and they're not very literate. They go to the doctor's and they get told they have to have this major surgery, they end up with a kidney missing and obviously the doctors have sold it on as transplants without the knowledge of the patients you see.

This reflects arguments in Chapters 2 and 3 about risk. Knowledge of risk, as Giddens (1991b) argues, leads to a distrust of expertise and a potential deconstruction of the lay–expert relationship. Some women within the study had even had bad family experiences leading to fatal consequences with health care in India. This had in the long run put them off. In talking about her fears about using health care within India, Kishwar drew on family experience:

The hygienic side of things is not very good and from the cases about which I hear, they don't sterilize their tools like we do and with AIDS going round. With somebody actually contracting AIDS, a family member

through that. It has put me off a bit, you know, using
health care there.

This was quite a common view among respondents, which
exemplifies their superficially paradoxical view of health care
products and services in India. Women within the study felt
pleased that they had access to health care in both Western
and non-Western contexts and felt that this gave them opportunities not open to other British populations. The women,
however, did see these opportunities through a lens of caution. Their desire to draw on such resources often related to
family and other contacts in India. In particular, this related
to whether these contacts had used various services before
and whether they had family or friends who were medical
practitioners in India. In contrast to the story of one of
Shahnaz's family members outlined earlier, most women
quite often felt that health care was better in the United Kingdom, with better-qualified staff and better facilities. Many
women within the study related mistrust to particular geographical areas of India, and said their use of health care
there depended on what area they were in. Meade, Horin,
and Gesler (1988) argue that, as with health care in many
geographical locations, India's heterogeneity and plurality
of health care results in spatial and social imbalance in the
quantity and quality of available health care. Regional differences in health care system mixes and health outcomes
create huge inequalities in health care delivery systems, and
this was reflected in the women's accounts.

Within the study many respondents used health products
and care within India. Respondents drew mostly (although
not exclusively) on Western remedies in India. Some women
within the study used these only in times of necessity when
visiting India. Others went to India specifically for treatments.
In the case of one respondent, Shahnaz, health care in India
was used when health care in the United Kingdom proved ineffective. Within the study, women also drew on non-Western
remedies in India, although this was to a lesser extent, highlighting their overall syncretic use of remedies within India.

Again, respondents' position as British Asians is a position more dynamic than one located statically between two cultures. Through their position as British Asians, women within the study have access to a plurality of remedies that they draw on syncretically. As members of a mobile group women within the study have access to diasporic networks in differing contexts. Such access is then fostered through processes inherent within globaliztion. Through such connections and processes women within the study are able to draw on discourses within (and between) India and Britain syncretically, making imagined connections with diasporas in other contexts (and homelands) become real. It is to some of the respondents' "other" diasporic connections that I will now turn.

CONNECTING THE SOUTH ASIAN DIASPORA: SYNCRECY IN OTHER CONTEXTS

The South Asian diaspora, argues Ghosh (1989), is oriented not so much to roots in a space–place and a desire to return, as to the ability to recreate culture in diverse locations. The transnational connections linking diaspora need not be articulated primarily through a real or symbolic homeland. Decentered lateral connections may be as important as those formed around a teleology of origin and return and a shared ongoing history of displacement; suffering, adaptation, or resistance may be as important as the projection of specific origin. Within this chapter I have talked about respondents' use of remedies in India. In discussing this, it is important to recognize that not all respondents share the same relationship to India. Women within the study were part of a broader decentralized Asian diaspora with connections in places like North America and backgrounds in East Africa, Europe, and other diasporic contexts. Several respondents, as argued earlier, had East African backgrounds; other respondents had Pakistani or Caribbean backgrounds. There were also those respondents with Indian backgrounds who had migrated from other European contexts to Britain. This spatial heritage influenced the respondents' use of remedies, both Western and non-Western, within India and other non-British locations. Within the study there was a split between women visiting India as if it were part of a "homeland" and those who felt like they were "foreigners" there. This tied in with respondents' identities in general and whether they saw themselves as British Asian women, as Indian women, as Muslim women, or as something else. The split was most keenly felt between those who had roots or family origins in East Africa, the Caribbean, or other parts of Europe and those families who were more directly from India. The latter on the whole were far more comfortable with visiting India and using health care there. This did not automatically stop those from other countries using health care in India, and in fact they were more likely to do so than to use health care in countries from which their families or they originally came. For instance, Rambha, who migrated to the United Kingdom from East Africa when she was three, talked about her feelings for East Africa and India:

> No, we haven't been back to East Africa, not for anything really. Health care there is very different. We used to live in a village where Madwani [the sugar plantation owner] ruled the whole village like and he, he provided the health service for all his workers and all the people who lived in the village worked for him anyway so . . . he's still got it going, the plantation, but I never go back, particularly not for health, oh no. I do visit India though, quite regularly.

This also translated to respondents' health choices. While women from East Africa felt comfortable using health care in India and transferred syncretic health goods between India and the United Kingdom, they were less likely to visit India specifically for health reasons. They were also less likely to draw on non-Western and syncretic remedies while visiting India. As Reena, another East African respondent, shows,

Oh, well I would use health care in India but only if I really had to, you know. I mean way back we have family there but I don't really know them. I definitely wouldn't use non-Western care there.

This mostly relates to differences between respondents of East African and Indian origin. As Jeffers, Hoggett, and Harrison (1996) argue, the East African Asian population in Leicester marks its difference from other Asian populations in Britain. They argue that the East African Asian community had by virtue of the particular colonial role it played in East African history become partially anglicized. The difference in respondents' accounts may relate to this. However, I would argue that the respondents' accounts also reflect Worsley's (1997) argument that certain elements of culture are spatially diverse and that this affects health choice. He gives the example of religion and argues that Hindus everywhere are assumed to subscribe to the same religious beliefs and the same medical theories. But, for example, Ayurveda in India differs from Ayurveda in Sri Lanka; doctors practice different parts and interpret texts differently. It is interesting to note within this study that women with East African backgrounds were both Hindu and Muslim, while respondents with backgrounds in the Indian subcontinent were Hindu, Muslim, and Sikh. This highlights the way in which variables of influence on health choices were spatially located. In contrast to the respondents with East African backgrounds, Charlotte, the respondent from the Caribbean, had very different views. She did visit Trinidad frequently and identified it as home, even though she had lived in Britain from the age of five. This respondent was also committed to herbal remedies in general, and alternatives and spiritual remedies, and visited the Caribbean to use these remedies:

In the Caribbean as well we have a lot of things, yeah there are a lot of things that we use, just simple things like ginger tea and it really works, a lot of root substances are good for getting rid of allergies and colds or keeping them at bay anyway. Oh I love to go back so I can use all these things. I just wish I could be there more often.

Within the study respondents had many connections with Asians in India as well as with members of the "decentralized" Asian diaspora in other contexts. As argued, for many of the women within the study their syncretic use of remedies was opened up cross-nationally from their context in Leicester to India. This opening up of syncrecy, however, was not a uniform process. Respondents with East African backgrounds in particular were less likely to draw on syncretic remedies within either East Africa or India. While they were more likely to visit India than East Africa, they were less likely than other respondents to do so for health reasons.

CONCLUSION

This chapter has focused primarily on the significance of geographical location, space, and globalization on the health choices of women within the study. Within the chapter geographical location has been seen as a key variable in understanding health choices. As the findings of the research have shown, the influence of the women's location in Leicester, a highly multicultural city, is significant. The influence of the two-way process of globalization emphasized by Friedman (1994) is also highlighted. The tension between the local and the global can be seen through women's movement (and use) of products in India, along with the circulation and access to health goods within their local context of Leicester. Globalization theorists have highlighted the ways in which globalization cannot be seen merely as cultural homogenization (Hall 1992b) nor cultural decentralization (Friedman 1994). The women's accounts are testimony to this through their emphasis on the interplay between cultural identity and global market forces, between local and global processes, and between consumption and cultural strategies.

The significance of both ethnicity and generation on health choice are highlighted within the chapter. The women's position as British Asians widens their access to a plurality of medicines in a diverse range of locations. As British Asians, women are socialized within Britain and within a wider globally dispersed diasporic network. This gives women equal access to both Western and non-Western medicines. Globalization further opens routes for diasporic groups, enhancing connections to an "imagined homeland" and to other diasporic contexts. Such processes enabled women within the study to move goods transculturally and to utilize health care and products in India. Ethnic group membership, generational positioning, and the processes inherent in globalization thus give rise to a variety of geographical spaces of health. Such spaces are less obtainable to other non-Asian British people. Alongside these processes, the overall growth of alternative medicine can also be seen to play a role in influencing health choices. Here, in particular, such growth can be seen to influence women's use of other non-Asian, non-Western remedies.

Broadly speaking, the discussion within this chapter highlights the need for globally dynamic and processual approaches to medical pluralism. Medical pluralism is built upon multiple transnational networks, networks that can be regionally situated but transcend national boundaries. As argued in the conclusion of this book, this is something worth exploring within new research, focusing on different diasporas in other national and international contexts. In the final chapter of this book the findings of the study as a whole will be evaluated, and the implications of the findings for research and policy in the areas of gender, ethnicity, and health will be discussed.

Chapter 6

Conclusion

This book has explored the influence of ethnicity, gender, and generation on the health choices of British Asian mothers. In today's global climate we find ourselves free to draw syncretically on all kinds of health products and services. At the start of this book the question was asked: What constitutes and constrains such syncrecy? How do ethnicity, gender, and generation affect access to and use of a plurality of health goods and systems? Drawing on empirical research with British Asian mothers, this book has explored the various ways in which health choices are characterized by a mix and match of different types of medicine. It has also looked at the influences behind these health choices. This book has illustrated the ways in which health choices vary according to contextual and material circumstances. In particular, within this study women's health choices related to particular types of illnesses, to their families, ethnic communities, and religions, to their location in Leicester, and to their access to a broader South Asian diasporic network. As shown throughout, these contextual circumstances intersect with women's ethnic, generational, and gendered identities and positions.

In drawing together and evaluating the aims and findings of this book, the conclusion will be split into three sections.

The first and main body of the conclusion will be concerned with the theory and findings of the study. The second section will reflect on the research process, also addressing the broader implications of the research. Finally, the third section will focus on potential trends within women's health choices and explore further uses of the theoretical framework.

THE SIGNIFICANCE OF
SYNCRECY AND CONTEXT

As shown throughout this book, the women's social and cultural contexts were central to their lives and significantly influenced their health choices. These contextual circumstances were interwoven with broader issues relating to ethnicity, gender, generation, and globalization. Explorations of such influences began in Chapter 2 with a focus on the significance of illness itself. The women's health choices were shown to be more syncretic regarding some illnesses and less so for others. Drawing on Cornwell's (1984) tripartite classification system, women's health choices could be seen to vary according to normal illness, health problems, and real illness. For general health problems the women's health choices tended to be weighted toward use of non-Western remedies, whereas the more serious conditions were, the more women were likely to use mostly Western medicines. Authors such as Giddens (1991a) question our faith in the expert systems of modern society; however, the women's accounts here showed a more complex picture. While the women were keen to use alternative medicine for normal illness and health problems, their faith ultimately lay in biomedicine regarding real illness. In highlighting the ways in which health choices were influenced by illness itself, the women's accounts have also highlighted the importance of social context on health choices. While the women's illnesses determined their health choices, these choices cannot be divorced from their geographical location, nor the strength of their social networks.

Chapter 3 focused on the influence of family, generation, and position within the life course. Drawing on the findings of the study, the chapter explored the ways in which women's health deteriorated after marriage. This supports earlier studies on women's health (M. Stacey 1985). In addition to influencing health status, marriage was shown to influence the women's health choices. Through husbands, women within the study engaged with new non-Western health remedies, which were by and large regarded by them as beneficial to their health. The women's accounts also highlighted a conflict between men and women over their children's health and the use of different remedies, and also the constraining roles of in-laws. When thinking about children's health, the women's choices were more complex. A moral status was ascribed to children's health. While alternative medicine was deemed more natural for children on the one hand, drawing on arguments made within Chapter 2 women ultimately deferred to Western biomedicine.

In particular, Chapter 3 highlighted the complex nature of the gender dynamic within the domestic sphere. Women asserted themselves within the domestic sphere through their choice of certain remedies for themselves and also as mediators of family health. They were, however, also constrained by marriage having a negative effect on their health status and men preventing them from using certain types of medicine on the children. It must be recognized that marriage stands as a contested domain for the women, suggesting that the findings require a more complex framework than that developed in previous research. Previous research on women's and men's health has focused mostly on measuring differentials in health status (Doyal 1995). While this is important, what is needed (as the research here shows) is a framework that looks not just at women's health status in comparison to their husbands but also explores husbands' influence on health choices and use of Western and non-Western medicine. The wider role of the family and children could also be included in such investigations.

Chapter 3 also emphasized the significance of age and generation, length of settlement, and position in the life course for health choices. Women within the study identified dif-

ferences in generation and health choices. They identified
their own parents' (particularly their mothers') health choices
as being located mostly within non-Western remedies. They
saw their own health choices as syncretic and their children's
as located mostly within Western remedies. Women also saw
themselves at a particular point in the life course, as mothers with dependent children. Most of the women felt that
their health choices had changed on becoming adults, getting married, and becoming mothers. As younger single
women they were much more likely to draw on Western remedies. They felt that this would change as they got older and
became grandmothers themselves. They felt that they would
be more likely to draw on non-Western remedies (Worsley
1997). Overall, the influence of family as explored within
Chapter 3 highlights the important intersection of generation
and ethnicity with location and globalization. The women,
as British Asians (a globally dispersed ethnic group), had
family members in a variety of geographical locations across
the globe. Globalization, with its emphasis on the deconstruction of borders and boundaries, helped foster these family
connections, making the influence of family on the women's
health choices local, national, and global.

Chapter 4 explored the influence of community and religion (both locally and globally) on the women's health
choices. Many health choices were associated with religious
rituals and there were differences between respondents of
differing religions. Community was also influential. Here the
focus was on what Ballard (1994, 29) calls "real" communities; that is, communities that are parochially organized as
opposed to the imagined "community" of India or diasporic
connections in other parts of the globe. Community within
women's accounts was heterogeneous and layered. The
women talked about different types of community, ranging
from identification with a particular religious community,
such as Muslim or Sikh, to identification with broader notions of an Asian community. The women also talked about
socializing with other communities, such as with White communities. In exploring the influence of religion and commu-

nity on health choices, Chapter 4 highlighted two key issues. First, it emphasized the heterogeneous nature of both religion and community. The women's accounts showed that there can be no such thing as a bounded sense of either religion or community. Both are context specific and shift over time. Second, it highlighted the ways in which the influence of religion and community were also gender and generationally specific. Whether in terms of friendship or community, the women mostly talked about the influence of other women on their health choices. Their generational position also informed their sense of community. Their position as British Asians enabled them to move in and out of different generational layers of community, capturing differing influences.

The women's sense of identity and how this influenced their health choices was also explored. Two strains of identity studies were bought together here. First, studies on second-generation migrants have in recent years focused on the complex sense of cultural location felt by such groups. Identity is seen as fluid and multiply located (Hall 1992). Second, studies on health have also recently turned to focus on a more narrative approach, exploring the ways in which people, when talking about health, also disclose information about themselves and their position within the social world (Radley and Billig 1996). Within the study women talked about the multifaceted nature of their identities, for instance, as British, Asian, Muslim, mothers, and daughters. They did, however, have an overall sense of themselves as British Asian women and saw this position as both influencing and reflecting their use of syncretic remedies. This highlights the significance of these two substantive strains of identity and brings together the women's sense of ethnic identity with their choices about health.

Finally, in Chapter 5 the influence of space, geographical location, and the reciprocal nature of globalization were explored. The women's accounts highlighted the importance of their location in Leicester, their connections and resources within India, the movement of health products between countries, and the use and access to health care in other Western and non-Western contexts. The women identified their location in Leicester as enabling them to have broad access to syncretic remedies. Many of the women had come to Leicester from other parts of the United Kingdom to marry, and felt that within Leicester they had access to remedies unavailable to them in other British contexts. The women's connections with India (and more minimally diasporas elsewhere) also geographically extended their access to a plurality of health remedies, both Western and non-Western.

These local–global connections are strengthened by (and reflect) processes inherent within globalization, fostering the transcultural flow of syncretic health goods and enabling the respondents' syncretic use of remedies in India. This opened up women's access to syncretic remedies in diverse locations. As argued, it also shifted connections between Britain and diasporas in various places and populations from "imagined" to "real." Again, the significant influence of the women's position as British Asians, as part of a mobile group with a significantly globally dispersed network, is highlighted. This position is a dynamic one that transcends "between two cultures" approaches by moving in and out of differing categories in different contexts. The spatial mapping of health choices must be seen to highlight the current phase of globalization. It reflects the reciprocal nature of the globalization process and marks an increased globalization of alternative medicine and ethnicity.

The significance of social context as shown throughout this book has emphasized the ways in which health choices cannot be seen as merely "free floating." As each chapter shows, health choices are deeply embedded in and informed by people's social and cultural contexts. These contextual influences are related to gender, generation, ethnic location, and globalization. The women's position as British Asians played a significant role in influencing health choices. Through membership in a particular ethnic group the women had access to a whole range of non-Western health remedies, both locally and globally. The process of globalization with its emphasis on the deconstruction of borders and boundaries fostered the women's contact with ethnic group members in other locations. The women's position as British born or having lived here since the age of five also gave them access to Western medicine that is often less accessible to older generations due to problems associated with linguistic barriers. Their gendered positions as mothers and mediators of family health further influenced their ability to make certain health choices. While health choices were relative to contextual and material circumstances and the respondents' position as British Asians, they were also temporally specific, changing over time. This highlights the important influence of age, length of settlement, and position within the life course on health choices.

LOCATING HEALTH CHOICES IN TIME

It is important to recognize that one can capture health choices only at a particular time and in particular contexts (Radley and Billig 1996). In Chapter 1 I argued that people do not simply "have" health choices in a fixed manner. Rather, like the process of identity construction itself (and as part of that identity construction), health choices are fluid and change over time. This is similar to Parsons's (1951) account of the "sick role." People take on the sick role (i.e., the social role of the sick person), but it is expected that people will move in and out of that role at particular times and contexts. Studies on migrant and minority beliefs about and use of plural medicine are located in particular temporal contexts. Studies capture health choices at only one moment in time, but acknowledge that these are fluid and vary as people pass through the life course (Kraut 1997). The intersection of time with contextual and material circumstances was influential on women's health choices. The findings highlighted a temporal quality to the women's health choices. The women's health choices were syncretic in particular contexts and also at particular times. In broader terms, this highlights the ways in which influences such as ethnicity, gender, generation, and globalization on our health choices cannot be seen as fixed, but rather are temporally located.

In Chapter 2 women's accounts of particular illnesses can be situated within a temporal framework. From the women's accounts it became important to recognize that while their health choices might be syncretic for particular illnesses, this cannot be fixed in time, as health choices changed over "illness time." The women may treat an illness in a particular way, drawing on syncretic remedies. If they failed to get better over time, then they would shift their use of remedies from one to another. This also often coincided with shifts in the women's accounts from their use of remedies mostly within the private realm to use of them mostly within the public realm. The women's attitudes to particular illnesses also might shift over time as they became more familiar with that illness, moving from using one type of discourse to another.

As shown in Chapter 3, when talking about family and life course women often talked about how health choices changed over time. While the women identified their health choices as syncretic during this particular phase of the life course, they had different projections for syncrecy in the future. Health choices might still be syncretic, but women within the study felt that they would draw more heavily on non-Western remedies when they got older. They seemed to have a clear sense of the impact of change, both generationally and as they progressed through the life course and were faced by different stresses and strains. As argued, generation was also a relevant dimension here. The women identified differences in the health choices of different generations over time. It appeared that the women's mothers' use of Asian remedies decreased, while theirs were syncretic and their children's orientations were mostly Western. These health choices were not fixed, but rather reflected family members' positions within the life course. It would be interesting to see how the women's health choices changed as they became older and became grandmothers themselves. Drawing on arguments in Chapter 4, religion, community, and identity can also be placed in a temporal framework. Identity itself is temporally located and through it the women's health choices were captured at a particular time, again reflecting their position as British Asian mothers. Religion and community influenced women's use of particular types of remedies at specific times. While religion seemed a constant influence on women's health choices in some way, they identified the influence of different aspects of community as changing over time. This does not suggest an "assimilation" approach, where the women's health choices were subject to Westernization over time. Rather, the women's position as British Asians enabled them to move in and out of different community positions, creating new spaces.

Finally, the importance of the intersection of time with space was highlighted in Chapter 5. The women's health choices were syncretic at particular times and in particular spaces. Space and time intersect in two different ways within the women's accounts, influencing health choices in a local–global sense. First, women's migration within the United Kingdom over time influenced their health choices. Second, the many processes associated with globalization, such as time–space compression and opening up of national boundaries, enabled the women to gain easy access to the Asian diaspora in other geographical contexts. This was reflected by shifts in the women's locations, and "real" and "imagined" communities becoming interchangeable at different times and in differing contexts. Both these local–global influences can be seen as timely qualities, as women use them syncretically over different times and spaces.

Such temporal specificity means that we can never pin down in any fixed manner what influences health choices. The social contexts within which we live change over time and such changes affect our health choices. The influence of ethnicity is subject to change in relation to shifts within our social world, and this in turn affects health choices. For the women within this study, and possibly for other members of migrant groups, health choices changed as people moved through different stages of migration and settlement.

As the women's accounts highlight, wider structural resources change both as a response to changes in our social contexts and in response to factors existing external to them. Again, such shifts affect health choices. For instance, access to certain provisions and state services may change according to material position and geographical location. Alternatively, wider health policies and transformations within the health services will also affect health choices. The fact that we cannot pin down and fix health choices does not make the process of exploring them any less valid. It is still important to capture the influence of contexts in order to compare patterns across groups over time and geographical context. It is also important to document key trends in order to identify areas for further research and policy attention.

REFLECTIONS AND IMPLICATIONS

The research on which this book is based aimed to address gaps within existing research in the areas of ethnicity, gender, generation, globalization, and health. The findings of the study not only address such gaps, but also have implications for future research and potentially address policy issues. One of the main aims of the study was to take up Eade's (1997) call for more qualitative research into migrant and minority health choices. The research in particular aimed to contribute to the small body of existing literature on the health choices of minority women. As noted in Chapter 1, the experiences of Black women have received little attention in the literature. We know that they are more likely than White women to be disadvantaged in terms of health in a range of identifiable ways (J. Douglas 1992), but there have been very few studies that have explored the health choices of Black women. Although there is a growing literature on "race," ethnicity, and health, gender has remained quite peripheral within this literature. Work on gender and health, on the other hand, has paid insufficient attention to ethnicity.

This book has highlighted the significance of conceptualizations of health and illness; family, generation, and life course; religion and community; and location and globalization for the women's health choices. In doing so it emphasizes the need to situate health choices within a framework that recognizes the importance of both culture and social structure. This supports Bayne-Smith's (1996) argument that the health of women from Black and ethnic minority groups cannot be separated from their roles as wives, mothers, daughters, sisters, employees, and community participants. Similarly, their experiences of morbidity and mortality cannot be understood outside the broader institutions of culture and social structure, such as the education system, housing provision, health and welfare services, religion, family patterns, and the economy. Overall, this study supports previous claims (J. Douglas 1998) that the health care needs of women from Black and minority ethnic communities need to be addressed strategically by policy makers, practitioners, and researchers. We need to see more translation of research into practice in health care provision. International connections highlighted within these research findings emphasize the need and feasibility of dissemination and exchange of information to women on an international level (Doyal 1995).

As noted in Chapter 1, Ahmad (1993) has identified two (both inadequate) approaches to the study of race, ethnicity, and health. The first involves large-scale epidemiological studies that singularly fail to get at perceptions of health and illness. The second is the culturalist approach, which locates health and illness purely within cultural explanations. Throughout this book, from developing the theoretical framework to reporting the findings of the study, the aim has been to transcend these two approaches. On the one hand, social and cultural explanations are taken into account where appropriate. However, the study has also been mindful of diversity, recognizing that social and cultural explanations should not be used in a way that imposes homogeneity on a group of people while ignoring variations in religion, ethnicity, class, and gender.

The need to take into account issues of cultural diversity also brings into question the very feasibility of research across difference. The difficulties of researching across difference and in particular racial difference were raised in Chapter 1. How could I as a White woman interview South Asian women? While the tensions of researching across difference can never truly be overcome, the book does highlight the possibilities of such research. Each chapter in its own way addresses the difficulties of researching "women's" health. Occasionally within the research I felt that women were unable to disclose certain types of information; for example, about issues such as racism within health services. Mostly, though, the women seemed to welcome the opportunity to talk in detail to someone about their health. Also, there were some shared experiences between myself and my respondents. I was around the same age as many of the women (mid-twenties), was from Leicester, and had been to India. While such commonalities did not (and cannot) overcome racial difference within the study, they certainly helped to build rapport and make such research more feasible. The study from this point of view attempted to avoid overgeneral universalism and overdetailed particularism. Rather than suggesting the unfeasibility of research on gender and difference, the research, through a "partial perspective" approach (Haraway 1988; Harding 1991) emphasizes the need to proceed with sensitivity.

From the outset, the aim of the study was to explore the health choices of women who had children. By focusing on the health of mothers, the research in particular wanted to pick up on findings of previous studies, which focused on the role of women as mediators of family health (Blaxter and Paterson 1982). As argued in Chapter 1, a prominent area of research regarding women's health has been women's activities as care givers, in families and in society at large, as primary consumers of health care for themselves and others (Graham 1984, 1993). Through focusing on women with children, I hoped that women's accounts would contain not just views about their own health but also that of their families, husbands, and children. The women did talk about the health choices of other members of their families, and it seemed that through talking more generally about family health the women were able to talk more about their own health. From the women's accounts it became apparent that women within the study were also the mediators of family health. In most cases women took on the major responsibility for their family's health. The women were also the major consumers of health care. This was the case even in differing contexts, when health products and health care were used in India. The women also quite often had negative perceptions of their own health in comparison to their husbands', which again is consistent with previous studies on gender differentials and health (Blaxter 1983).

The impact of generation on health choices of the British Asian women within the study was also a key aim. Little research has explored the importance of generation on migrant and minority health choices (Greenslade, Madden, and Pearson 1997; Kraut 1997). As argued earlier, studies on identity (e.g., Parker 1995) have focused on the unique identity of various diasporic groups born or raised in the West. In recent years they have moved away from the "between two cultures" approaches advocated by Watson (1977) to explore the syncretic, multiply located, and changing identity of this particular generation. It was the aim of this book to draw on these frameworks, applying them within a health context to look at the influence of generation and length of settlement on health choices and to explore the health choices of British Asian women within the study. This study supports arguments made in research on identity. The women's health choices were syncretic and this relates implicitly to their position as British Asians. Being part of this generational group, with both roots and routes in Asian and English culture, opened up access to both Western and non-Western remedies. Rather than being "between two cultures," the women actively engaged at differing times and in particular contexts with different cultures. This fostered a syncretic use of remedies that was fluid and multiply located, just like identity.

In Chapter 1 the exploration of health choices was situated within the wider context of debates on plural medicine.

A number of authors have shown how the use of alternative medicine has increased significantly in the last decade (Cant and Sharma 1999; West 1992). Worsley (1997) argues that many people in Britain, after consulting their GPs, feel dissatisfied with the symptom-oriented approach in Western medicine and turn to alternatives. Throughout the study the women's accounts reflected these trends. As argued, women's position as British Asians, as part of a particular ethnic and generational group, along with various contextual circumstances and broader global processes, influenced their syncretic use of remedies. This use can also be related to a general increase in lay use of alternative medicine. It is important to recognize that this influence relates mostly to the women's use of Asian medical remedies. Reflecting back on the typology of alternative medicine as outlined by Cant and Sharma (1999), we can recognize the diversity in the category "alternative." Within this study women also drew on a number of other alternative non-Asian remedies, and this reflects broader, more general trends in lay use of alternative medicine.

However, while the women's accounts emphasized a general increase in use of alternative medicine, they also highlighted limitations to this usage. Women would try remedies and use them on themselves and for general illness, but they ultimately deferred to Western biomedicine. This shows that while there is an increase to alternative medicine, this in no way poses a threat to the hegemonic position of Western biomedicine. Worsley (1997) points to the reciprocal movement of Western and non-Western health products, suggesting that although Western medicine diffuses pretty rapidly, the traffic is not all one way. What the findings of this study show is that while the traffic of health goods may not be all one way, the hegemony and status attributed to health systems still lie with biomedicine.

This book overall has highlighted the importance of health research on ethnicity, gender, generation, and plural medicine. The health needs of women, their consistent lower assessments of health, and their beliefs and experiences of health and health care need to be heard and explored. The women's accounts emphasized the need, perhaps, for a more significant integration of alternative health behaviors into mainstream health care systems. While we may see some support for alternative health within our local doctors' surgeries, this tends to be sporadic. It is also often centered around practices such as acupuncture or chiropractic, excluding other alternative systems (e.g., Ayurveda). As Finch and Groves (1983) argue, welfare structures have always depended on the unpaid work of women. The findings of this study concur with this. They continue to emphasize the ongoing need for welfare structures to support and take pressure off women's roles as mediators and care givers within the family. Gender differentials in health status were also reflected in the research findings. These point to a need for further research in the area and greater policy sensitivity toward such differentials. Within this context it would be useful to explore gendered differentials further by focusing on syncrecy in Asian men's health choices.

Much epidemiological research on ethnicity and health has lumped ethnic groups together. Research has failed to see the heterogeneity within ethnic groups, choosing instead to see them as homogenous entities from which generalizations about health can be made. As this study has shown, there are many differences within and between ethnic groups: differences by generation, religion, region of origin, and so on. By emphasizing this the book has highlighted the need for future epidemiological studies in both the United Kingdom and the United States on ethnicity and health to be sensitive in their categorization of women from ethnic minority groups. The diversity of health experiences among South Asian women within this study suggests a need to diversify categories of research. This would enable research to capture more broadly women's health needs. Policy and research, in developing ways to approach and increase good health and well-being, should also take heed of the significant influence of generational differences. The findings of this study highlight the importance of intergenerational research and show the differences in health needs between generations, enabling us to see which populations are in particular need and deserve to be targeted. The study also opens up new possibilities, paving the way for further intergenerational research, which I will explore in the final section of this chapter. Finally, the need for more research in lay increases in the use of plural medicine is apparent throughout this book. Such approaches will need to be globally dynamic and processual and emphasize the argument that pluralism is built upon multiple, transnational networks that can be regionally situated but transcend national boundaries.

THE TRANSFORMATION OF SYNCRECY

The theoretical framework has been useful for exploring the health choices of women within the context of this study. In areas other than health the concept of syncrecy has also proved useful. As Holton (1998) argues, in terms of issues of cultural identity the very fluidity of syncretic cultural forms is important to sustaining identity in an epoch of globalization. In talking about syncretism and world music, he argues that music and its rituals can be used to create a model whereby identity can be understood neither as a fixed essence nor as a vague and utterly contingent construction to be reinvented by the will. This is a useful concept and framework, but we need to ask whether it has limitations. While recognizing that syncrecy is useful for exploring many issues within this phase of globalization in varying contexts, is it a concept with which we can generalize? In looking at identity in various parts of the global field, ethnic and other kinds of cultural boundaries are being reerected to the point of promotion or enforcing purity by various means. For example, support remains for bounded primordial constructions of cultural identity among both White and Black, Western and non-Western. This highlights the limitations and specificity of the term. On the other hand, some writers suggest terms such as "hybridity" and "syncrecy" are too generalizable. Baucon (1996) argues that in a world in which we inevitably discover that everything is "hybrid" (as it is in his vision), we might as well close up shop.

I would argue, however, that the beauty and potential of the framework of syncrecy lies in its creation of a tension between these two approaches. Syncrecy does allow for tension between the universal and the particular, between the personal and the social, between the local and the global. This is why the term has been so helpful in the context of this particular study. This tension is always changing and is processual. In this sense syncrecy is rather like a dialectic process itself, as the accounts of the women researched here show. For instance, at times certain types of medicines are privileged within the womens' accounts, sometimes Western medicine over non-Western. At other times the findings show there might be significant commonalities across Western and non-Western remedies. The framework of syncrecy can be seen, therefore, as fluid and polyvocal, allowing for plurality. There is both commonality and contradiction within the framework, and the women's accounts suggest that at particular times and in particular contexts remedies come to be held in tension with one another. Does this mark an end point to syncrecy? Do categories eventually merge? I would suggest not; syncrecy will not necessarily be transcended and replaced by a new, more advanced "synthesis" of remedies that merge together. It is also unlikely that a move away from syncrecy to focus on just one type of medicine would provide an adequate framework.

To go back to Fitzpatrick's (1984) argument at the start of this book, health choices will always be syncretic in the sense that they will continue to be drawn from distinct and disparate sources. Syncrecy in this sense will continue to be a useful framework. However, as work on the Black Atlantic by Gilroy (1993) highlights, syncretic forms are never repeated in the same way, but are contextually specific. The importance of this specificity is emphasized by viewing syncrecy as a dialectical process. As a dialectical process, syncrecy offers an analytical framework, not a chronological one. As highlighted in this book, it is rooted in the contexts of the women's lives. Earlier syncrecy was shown to be influenced by the women's gender, generation, and ethnicity at a particular time and within particular circumstances. Therefore, it must be recognized that the type of syncrecy will change according to historical, local, and personal context (Reed 1998; Schrijvers 1993).

Such contextualization of syncrecy directly addresses both sides of the critique that suggests that syncrecy is both too particularistic on the one hand and too generalizable on the other. Rather than being overspecific or overgeneralizable, syncrecy can assist with avoiding both of these problems. It is a transportable framework, but only once it has been contextualized. It can be exported, but in a form relevant to context. Syncrecy therefore has the potential to be "transformed" and used again in various contexts, although not in the form taken within this study. The use of non-Western and Western remedies syncretically by the women within this research will not be repeated in quite the same way by other groups. Within future research undertaken with other respondents, syncrecy will be reworked and reinscribed differently according to context. By adopting this dynamic and processual dialectical framework it is possible to explore more fully the potential use of syncrecy as a theoretical framework in various contexts. The rest of the conclusion will be concerned with asking several questions: What kinds of patterns do we think might occur within the women's health choices in the future? Will they still be syncretic? Can the theoretical framework be used further in other empirical contexts; for instance, for future generations and in different geographical contexts?

What will happen to the women's health choices? How might they change as the women progress throughout the life course and contextual circumstances alter? Will their health choices still be syncretic? While women within the study showed their ultimate faith lay in Western biomedicine, many of the women within the study did talk about their increased use of non-Western remedies as they got older and progressed through the life course. This can also be related to the wider trends toward increases in availability and use of alternative medicine by lay populations (Cant and Sharma 1999; Worsley 1997). Certainly, if recent media coverage highlighting the incompetence of biomedical doctors is anything to go by, we should come to expect a dramatic increase in lay use of alternative medicine. However, this can also be placed within the women's accounts alongside the increasing need, in light of hectic lifestyles, to draw on quick-fix solutions to health problems. Bearing this tension in mind, I would suggest that the women's health choices will continue to be syncretic, but that this syncrecy will be reworked and reinscribed as women's circumstances change. As for the continued influence of the women's position as British Asians, this is difficult to predict. While the women's accounts highlight changes over time in their position, this does not relate to a position of increased assimilation. Rather, the women seem to suggest an active engagement with categories of West and non-West, moving in and out of each at different times and contexts. On the one hand the women appeared to be moving toward drawing more on non-Western remedies advocated by their mothers, while at the same time they were being influenced by younger generations and other populations and communities. Again, this suggests a continuance of a dynamic position drawing on a number of remedies and going beyond a location "between two cultures."

Can the framework of syncrecy be exported to explore the health choices of others? This book has highlighted the use of the framework for British Asian women in Leicester. What about younger generations of Asian women who will have been more exposed to Western culture? The women's accounts suggested clear differences in syncretic use of remedies between generations. Women with teenage children often talked about how their children's health choices were more likely to be located within Western medicine. Is this likely to change as they become older and mothers themselves? In order to answer this question fully, additional empirical work would need to be conducted exploring the health choices of women in subsequent generations. This would take an exploration of the framework one step further. As shown, the concept of syncrecy is a more appropriate way of capturing the dynamic and fluid positioning of British Asian women within this study than the "between two cultures" approach advocated by Watson (1977). However, is syncrecy itself a phase; is it a way of coping in this particular era, as Holton (1998) argues? Or are there aspects of syncrecy relevant for subsequent generations, in particular as they themselves grow older? In what ways does syncrecy change?

A second issue worth exploring would be to see how geographically transportable the concept of syncrecy is. Many women within the study came from other parts of Britain, mostly Blackburn, Birmingham, and London. They alluded to differences in access to various remedies and talked about an increased use of non-Western medicine on moving to Leicester. It would be useful to explore the health choices of British Asian women within other regional contexts. Does the concept of syncrecy translate to other contexts within Britain? Similarly, this could be transposed cross-nationally. Gilroy (1993) talks about the Black Atlantic as an intercultural transnational formation linking Blacks in the United Kingdom and France as well as those in the United States and the Caribbean. This is a formation that is intermediate between the global and the local, and which has a dynamic history in which slavery, colonization, and migration all play parts. As argued within this study women talked about connections with Asian diasporas in other contexts. Again, it would be worth exploring these connections through studies of the Asian diaspora in America, Africa, Europe, and elsewhere to see how syncrecy compares. As Gilroy (1993) argues, while the Black Atlantic is transnational and transcultural, it generates local manifestations that are not identical to one another, but are reworked and reinscribed differently in different contexts. Is this the case for syncrecy in the health choices of Asian women in the United States?

Drawing on empirical research with British Asian mothers in Leicester, this book has highlighted the ways in which health choices are guided by ethnicity, gender, and generation. This book has looked at the syncretic nature of the choices, focusing on the ways in which these choices are embedded within the social context of the women's lives. In particular, this book has emphasized the significant influence of ethnicity on health choices. With the increased availability of globalization we are all faced by a plurality of health choices. However, as the women's accounts have shown throughout, for those who are members of a globally dispersed ethnic group, health choices are broadened, and those products available in the global marketplace can be transported and filtered through local contexts. The framework of syncrecy has captured such health choices, allowing for such local and global possibilities, and we should consider extending this further in explorations of health choices. In assessing the continued relevance of a postcolonial conceptual framework, Mani (1992) has argued that concepts and frameworks such as this must be adequately localized before extending or exporting them. Within the context of this study, the conceptual framework of syncrecy has been adequately localized, and it can now be extended and exported. We can then see if and in what ways syncrecy has a broad relevance in different personal, social, and historical contexts.

Bibliography

Ahmad, W.I.U. (Ed.). (1993). *Race and Health in Contemporary Britain*. Buckingham: Open University Press.

Ahmad, W.I.U. (1996). The trouble with culture. In D. Kelleher and S. Hillier (Eds.), *Researching Cultural Differences in Health*. London: Routledge.

Alexander, C. (1996). *The Art of Being Black: The Creation of Black British Youth Identities*. Oxford: Clarendon Press.

Anderson, B. (1991). *Imagined Communities: Reflections on the Origin and Spread of Nationalism*. London: Verso.

Anderson, M. L. (1993). Studying across difference: Race, class and gender in qualitative research. In J. H. Stanfield and R. M. Dennis (Eds.), *Race and Ethnicity in Research Methods*. London: Sage.

Andrews, L., Lokuge, S., Sawyer, M., Martin, J., Lilywhite, L., and Kennedy, D. (1998). The use of alternative therapies by children with asthma: A brief report. *Journal of Paediatrics, 34*, 131–134.

Annandale, E. (1998). *The Sociology of Health and Medicine: A Critical Introduction*. Cambridge: Polity Press.

Appadurai, A. (1990) Disjuncture and difference in the global cultural economy. In M. Featherstone (Ed.), *Global Culture*. London: Sage.

Apter, T. (1990). *Altered Loves: Mothers and Daughters During Adolescence*. New York: Facade Columbine.

Arber, S. (1997). Comparing inequalities in women's and men's health in Britain in the 1990's. *Social Science and Medicine, 44*, 773–788.

Armstrong, D., and Pierce, M. (1996). Afro-Caribbean lay beliefs about diabetes: An exploratory study. In S. Hillier and D. Kelleher (Eds.), *Researching Cultural Differences in Health.* London: Routledge.

Back, L. (1993). Gendered participation: Masculinity and fieldwork in a South London community. In D. Bell, P. Caplan, and W. J. Karim (Eds.), *Gendered Fields: Women, Men and Ethnography.* London: Routledge.

Ballard, R. (1994). *Desh Pardesh: The South Asian Presence in Britain.* London: Hurst.

Baucon, I. (1996). Charting the "Black Atlantic." In *Postmodern Culture.* Retrieved from: <http://www.jefferson.village.Virginia.EDU/pmc/current.issue/baucon.997.html>. Last accessed 1998.

Bausinger, H. (1990). *Folk Culture in a World of Technology.* Bloomington: Indiana University Press.

Bayne-Smith, M. (1996). *Race, Gender and Health.* London: Sage.

Beck, L. C., Trombetta, W. L., and Share, S. (1986). Using focus group sessions before decisions are made. In *North Carolina Medical Journal, 47*, 73–74.

Beck, U. (1992). *Risk Society: Towards a New Modernity.* London: Sage.

Bernard, J. S. (1975). *Women, Wives and Mothers.* Chicago: Aldine.

Bhabha, H. (1992). *The Location of Culture.* London: Routledge.

Bhattacharya, D. P. (1986). *Paglami: Ethnopsychiatric Knowledge in Bengal* (Foreign and Comparative East Asian Studies no. 11). Syracuse, NY: Syracuse University Press, Maxwell School of Citizenship in Public Affairs.

Bhopal, K. (1999). South Asian women and arranged marriages in East London. In R. Barot, H. Bradley, and S. Fenton (Eds.), *Ethnicity, Gender and Social Change.* Basingstoke: Macmillan.

Blaxter, M. (1983). The causes of disease: Women talking. *Social Science in Medicine, 17*, 59–69.

Blaxter, M. (1990). *Health and Lifestyle.* London: Routledge.

Blaxter, M., and Paterson, E. (1982). *Mothers and Daughters: A Three Generational Study of Health Attitudes and Behaviours.* London: Heinemann.

Bogue, R. (1989). *Deleuze and Guattari*. London: Routledge.

Boon, H., Brown, J. B., Gavin, A., Kennard, M. A., and Stewart, M. (1999). Breast cancer survivors' perceptions of complementary/alternative medicine (CAM): Making the decision to use or not to use. *Qualitative Health Research, 9*, 639–653.

Bordo, S. (1990). Reading the slender body. In M. Jacobus, E. Fox-Keller, and S. Shuttleworth (Eds.), *Body/Politics: Women and the Discourses of Science*. London: Routledge.

Bowes, A., and Domokos, T. M. (1993). South Asian women and health services: A study in Glasgow. *New Community, 19*, 611–626.

Bowes, A., and Domokos, T. M. (1996). Pakistani women and maternity care: Raising muted voices. *Sociology of Health and Illness, 18*, 45–65.

Bowler, I. (1993). They're not the same as us: Midwives stereotypes of South Asian descent maternity patients. *Sociology of Health and Illness, 15*, 157–177.

Bradby, H. (1999). Negotiating marriage: Young Punjabi women's assessment of their individual and family interests. In R. Barot, H. Bradley, and S. Fenton (Eds.), *Ethnicity, Gender and Social Change*. Basingstoke: Macmillan.

Bradley, H. (1996). *Fractured Identities: Changing Patterns of Inequality*. Cambridge: Polity Press.

Brady, M., Kunitz, S., and Nash, D. (1997). Austrailian Aboriginies conceptualisations of health and the world health organisation. In M. Worboys and L. Markes (Eds.), *Migrants, Minorities and Health: Historical and Contemporary Studies*. London: Routledge.

Brannen, J., Dodd, K., Oakley, A., and Storey, P. (1994). *Young People, Health and Family Life*. Buckinghamshire: Open University Press.

Bridgen, M. L. (1995). Unproven (questionable) cancer therapies. *Western Journal of Medicine, 163*, 463–469.

British Holistic Medical Association. (1992). Response to the British Medical Association report. In M. Saks (Ed.), *Alternative Medicine in Britain*. Oxford: Clarendon Press.

British Medical Association. (1992). Report on alternative medicine. In M. Saks (Ed.), *Alternative Medicine in Britain*. Oxford: Clarendon Press.

Brown, G. W., and Harris, T. O. (1978). *The Social Origins of Depression*. London: Tavistock.

Bury, M. (1982). Chronic illness as biographical disruption. *Sociology of Health and Illness, 4*, 167–182.

Bury, M., and Holme, A. (1991). *Life after Ninety*. London: Routledge.

Busfield, J. (1996). *Men, Women and Madness: Understanding Gender and Mental Disorder*. Basingstoke: Macmillan.

Butler, J. (1993). *Bodies That Matter: On the Discursive Limits of Sex*. New York: Routledge.

Bystydzienski, J. M., and Resnik, E. P. (1994). *Women in Cross Cultural Transitions*. Bloomington, IN: Phi Delta Kappa Education Foundation.

Campbell, J. (1975a). Attribution of illness: Another double standard. *Journal of Health and Social Behaviour, 16*, 114–126.

Campbell, J. (1975b). The child in the sick role: Contributions of age, sex, parental status and parental values. *Journal of Health and Social Behaviour, 19*, 35–51.

Cant, S., and Calnan, M. (1991). On the margins of the medical marketplace? An exploratory study of alternative practitioners perceptions. *Sociology of Health and Illness, 13*, 34–51.

Cant, S., and Sharma, U. (1999). *A New Medical Pluralism? Alternative Medicine, Doctors, Patients and the State*. London: UCL Press.

Carter, E. (1984). Alice in the consumer wonderland: West German case studies in gender and consumer culture. In A. McRobbie and M. Nava (Eds.), *Gender and Generation*. Hampshire: Macmillan.

Chamberlain, M. (1981). *Old Wives Tales: Their History, Remedies and Spells*. London: Virago.

Charles, N., and Walters, V. (1998). Age and gender in women's accounts of their health: Interviews with women in South Wales. *Sociology of Health and Illness, 20*, 331–350.

Chhachhi, S., and Price, J. (1998). Raktpushp (Blood flower). In M. Shildrick and J. Price (Eds.), *Vital Signs: Feminist Reconfigurations of the Bio/logical Body*. Edinburgh: Edinburgh University Press.

Clifford, J. (1997). *Routes: Travel and Translation in the Late Twentieth Century*. Cambridge: Harvard University Press.

Clifford, J., and Marcus G. (1986). *Writing Culture: The Poetics and Politics of Ethnography*. Berkeley and Los Angeles: University of California Press.

Cornwell, J. (1984). *Hard Earned Lives: Accounts of Health and Illness from East London*. London: Tavistock.

Crow, G., and Allan, G. (1994). *Community Life: An Introduction to Local Social Relations.* Hemel Hempstead: Harvester Wheatsheaf.

Currer, C. (1986). Concepts of mental well- and ill-being: The case of pathan mothers in Britain." In C. Currer and M. Stacey (Eds.), *Concepts of Health, Illness and Disease: A Comparative Perspective.* Leamington Spa: Berg.

Davey, B., Gray, A., and Seale, C. (Eds.). (1995). *Health and Disease: A Reader.* Buckingham: Open University Press.

Davis, K. (1997). *Embodied Practices: Feminist Perspectives on the Body.* London: Sage.

Donovan, J. (1986). *We Don't Buy Sickness, It Just Comes: Health, Illness and Health Care in the Lives of Black People in London.* Gower: Aldershot.

Douglas, J. (1992). Black women's health matters: Putting black women back on the research agenda. In H. Roberts (Ed.), *Women's Health Matters.* London: Routledge.

Douglas, J. (1998). Meeting the health needs of women from black and minority ethnic communities. In L. Doyal (Ed.), *Women and Health Services.* Buckinghamshire: Open University Press.

Douglas, M. (1986). *Risk Acceptability According to the Social Sciences.* London: Routledge.

Doyal, L. (1995). *What Makes Women Sick: Gender and the Political Economy of Health.* Basingstoke: Macmillan.

Drefus, H., and Rabinow, P. (1982). *Michel Foucault: Beyond Structuralism and Hermeneutics.* Harvester: Brighton.

Dwyer, K. (1991). *Arab Voices: The Human Rights Debate in the Middle East.* London: Routledge.

Eade, J. (1997). The power of the experts: The plurality of beliefs and practices concerning health and illness among Bangladeshis in Tower Hamlets, London. In L. Marks and M. Worboys (Eds.), *Migrants, Minorities and Health: Historical and Contemporary Studies.* London: Routledge.

Espiritu, Y. (1992). *Asian American Panethnicity: Bridging Institutions and Identities.* Philadelphia: Temple University Press.

Featherstone, M. (1991). *Consumer Culture and Postmodernism.* London: Sage.

Fenton, S., and Sadiq-Sangster, A. (1996). Culture, relativism and the expression of mental distress: South Asian women in Britain. *Sociology of Health and Illness, 18,* 66–85.

Fernando, S. (1991). *Mental Health, Race and Culture*. Basingstoke: Macmillan.

Finch, J., and Groves, A. (1983). *A Labour of Love: Women, Work and Caring*. London: RKP.

Fitzpatrick, R. (1984). Lay concepts of health and illness. In R. Fitzpatrick, J. Hinton, S. Newman, G. Scrambler, and J. Thompson (Eds.), *The Experience of Illness*. London: Tavistock.

Ford, G. 1988. Science and ideology: The Marxist perspective. In Z. Sardar (Ed.), *The Revenge of Athena: Science, Exploitation and the Third World*. London: Mansell.

Foucault, M. (1972). *Archaeology of Knowledge*. London: Tavistock.

Fox, N. (1993). *Postmodernism, Sociology and Health*. Buckinghamshire: Open University Press.

Frankenburg, R., and Mani, L. (1996). Crosscurrents, crosstalk: Race, "postcoloniality," and the politics of location. In S. Lavie and T. Swedenburg (Eds.), *Displacement, Diaspora and Geographies of Identity*. Durham, NC: Duke University Press.

Friedman, J. (1994). *Cultural Identity and Global Process*. London: Sage.

Frith, S. (Ed.). (1989). *World Music, Politics and Social Change*. Manchester: Manchester University Press.

Furnham, A., and Smith, C. (1988). Choosing alternative medicine: A comparison of the beliefs of patients visiting a general practitioner and a Homeopath. *Social Science and Medicine, 26*, 685–689.

Gardner, K. (1990). *Jumbo Jets and Paddy Fields: Migration and Village Life in Sylhet*. Unpublished doctoral dissertation, University of London.

Gardner, K. (1993). Mullahs, migrants, miracles: travel and transformation in Sylhet. *Contributions to Indian Sociology, 27*, 213–235.

Gardner, K. (1995). *Global Migrants, Local Lives*. London: Oxford University Press.

Geertz, C. (1993). *The Interpretation of Cultures: Selected Essays*. London: Fontana.

Ghosh, A. (1989). The diaspora in Indian culture. *Public Culture, 2*, 73–78.

Giddens, A. (1991a). *The Consequences of Modernity*. Cambridge: Polity Press.

Giddens, A. (1991b). *Modernity and Self Identity: Self and Society in the Late Modern Age*. Cambridge: Polity Press.

Gidoomal, R. (1993). *Sari 'N' Chips*. Surrey: South Asian Concern.

Gilroy, P. (1993). *The Black Atlantic: Double Consciousness and Modernity*. Cambridge: Harvard University Press.

Glaser, B. G., and Strauss, A. L. (1967). *The Discovery of Grounded Theory: Strategies for Qualitative Research*. London: Weiden Field and Nicolson.

Goldberg, D. (1993). *Racist Culture*. Oxford: Blackwell.

Graham, H. (1984). *Women, Health and the Family*. Sussex: Wheatsheaf.

Graham, H. (1985). Providers, negotiators and mediators: Women as the hidden carers. In E. Lewin and V. Oleson (Eds.), *Women, Health and Healing: Toward a New Perspective*. London: Tavistock.

Graham, H. (1993). *Hardship and Health in Women's Lives*. London: Harvester Wheatsheaf.

Graham, H., and Oakley, A. (1986). Competing ideologies of reproduction: Medical and maternal perspectives on pregnancy. In C. Currer and M. Stacey (Eds.), *Concepts of Health, Illness and Disease: A Comparative Perspective*. Leamington Spa: Berg.

Greenslade, L., Madden, M., and Pearson, M. (1997). From visible to invisible: The "problem" of the health of Irish people in Britain. In L. Marks and M. Worboys (Eds.), *Migrants, Minorities and Health: Historical and Contemporary Studies*. London: Routledge.

Grewal, I., and Kaplan, C. (1994). Introduction: Transnational feminist practices and questions of postmodernity. In I. Grewal and C. Kaplan (Eds.), *Scattered Hegemonies: Postmodernity and Transnational Feminist Practice*. Minneapolis: University of Minnesota Press.

Griffin, C. (1989). I'm not a women's libber but. . . . Feminism, consciousness and identity. In S. Skevington and D. Baker (Eds.), *The Social Identity of Women*. London: Sage.

Guo, Z. (2000). *Ginseng and Aspirin: Healthcare Alternatives for Aging Chinese in New York*. New York: Cornell University Press.

Gupta, O. K., and Gupta, S. O. (1985–1986). A study of the influence of American culture on the child-rearing attitudes of Indian mothers. *Indian Journal of Social Work, 46*, 95–104.

Hahlo, K. (1998). *Communities, Networks and Ethnic Politics*. Aldershot: Ashgate.

Hall, S. (1992a). New ethnicities. In J. Donald and A. Rattanansi (Eds.), *Race, Culture and Difference*. London: Sage.

Hall, S. (1992b). The question of cultural identity. In S. Hall, D. Held, and T. McGrew (Eds.), *Modernity and Its Futures*. Buckingham: Open University Press.

Hall, S., and Du Gay, P. (Eds.). (1996). *Questions of Cultural Identity*. London: Sage.

Hammersley, M. (1992). *What's Wrong with Ethnography*. London: Routledge.

Handler, R. (1986). Authenticity. *Anthropology Today, 2*, 2–5.

Hannerz, U. (1989). Notes on the Global Ecumene. *Public Culture, 1*, 66–75.

Haraway, D. (1988). Situated knowledge's: The science question in feminism and the privilege of the partial perspective. *Feminist Studies, 14*, 575–600.

Harding, S. (1987). *Feminism and Methodology*. Milton Keynes: Open University Press.

Harding, S. (1991). *Whose Science, Whose Knowledge?* Ithaca, NY: Cornell University Press.

Harris, L. (1993). Postmodernism and utopia: An unholy alliance. In M. Cross and M. Keith (Eds.), *Racism, the City and the State*. London: Routledge.

Helman, C. (1978). Feed a cold, starve a fever: Folk models of infection in an English suburban community, and their relation to medical treatment. *Culture, Medicine and Psychiatry, 2*, 107–137.

Herzlich, C. (1973). *Health and Illness*. London: Academic Press.

Hillier, S., and Rahman, S. (1996). Childhood development and behavioural and emotional problems as perceived by Bangladeshi parents in East London. In D. Kelleher and S. Hillier (Eds.), *Researching Cultural Differences in Health*. London: Routledge.

Hollway, W. (1989). *Subjectivity and Method in Psychology: Gender, Meaning and Science*. London: Sage.

Holton, R. J. (1998). *Globalization and the Nation-State*. Basingstoke: Macmillan.

Homans, H. (1985). Discomforts in pregnancy: Traditional remedies and medical prescriptions. In H. Homans (Ed.), *The Sexual Politics of Reproduction*. Aldershot: Gower.

Hyden, L.-C. (1997). Illness and narrative. *Sociology of Health and Illness, 19*, 48–69.

James, A. G. (1974). *Sikh Children in Britain*. London: Oxford University Press.

Jeffers, S., Hoggett, P., and Harrison, L. (1996). Race, ethnicity and community in three localities. *New Community, 22*, 111–126.

Jones, L. (1994). *The Social Context of Health Work*. Basingstoke: Macmillan.

Karseras, P., and Hopkins, E. (1987). *British Asians: Health in the Community*. Hampshire: Chichester.

Kelleher, D. (1996). A defence of the use of the terms ethnicity and culture. In D. Kelleher and S. Hillier (Eds.), *Researching Cultural Differences in Health*. London: Routledge.

Kelleher, D., and Islam, S. (1996). How should I live? Bangladeshi people and non-insulin dependent diabetes. In D. Kelleher and S. Hillier (Eds.), *Researching Cultural Differences in Health*. London: Routledge.

Kelly, M., and Field, D. (1996). Medical sociology, chronic illness and the body. *Sociology of Health and Illness, 18*, 241–257.

Khan, V. S. (1977). The Pakistanis: Mirpuri villagers at home and in Bradford. In J. Watson (Ed.), *Between Two Cultures*. Oxford: Blackwell.

Kirchstein, R. (1991). Research on women's health. *American Journal of Public Health, 81*, 291–293.

Kleinman, A. (1980). *Patients and Healers in the Context of Culture*. Berkeley and Los Angeles: University of California Press.

Knight, K. (2000). *The Catholic Encyclopedia*. Retrieved from: <http://www.newadvent.org/cathen/09703b.htm>. Last accessed Summer 2000.

Kraut, A. (1997). Southern Italian immigration to the US at the turn of the century and the perennial problem of the medicalised prejudice. In L. Marks and M. Worboys (Eds.), *Migrants, Minorities and Health: Historical and Contemporary Studies*. London: Routledge.

Lambert, H., and Sevak, L. (1996). Is cultural difference a useful concept? In D. Kelleher and S. Hillier (Eds.), *Researching Cultural Differences in Health*. London: Routledge.

Leder, D. (1990). *The Absent Body*. Chicago: Chicago University Press.

Leicester City Council. (1991a). *Census: Electoral Wards Profiles (City)*. Leicester: Leicester City Council.

Leicester City Council. (1991b). Leicester Key Facts: Ethnic Minorities. In *1991 Census*. Leicester: Leicester City Council.

Leslie, C. (1992). Interpretations of illness: Syncretism in modern Ayurveda. In C. Leslie and A. Young (Eds.), *Paths to Asian Medical Knowledge*. Berkeley and Los Angeles: University of California Press.

Loue, S. (1999). *Gender, Ethnicity and Health Research*. New York: Kluwer Academic/Plenum.

Macintyre, S. (1996). Gender differences in health. *Social Science and Medicine, 42*, 617–624.

Mama, A. (1995). *Beyond the Masks: Race, Gender and Subjectivity*. London: Routledge.

Mani, L. (1992). Cultural theory, colonial texts: Reading eyewitness accounts of widow burning. In L. Grossberg, C. Nelson, and P. Treichler (Eds.), *Cultural Studies*. New York: Routledge.

Marcus, G. (1992). Past, present and emergent identities: Requirements for ethnographies of the late twentieth century modernity worldwide. In S. Lash and J. Friedman (Eds.), *Modernity and Identity*. Oxford: Basil Blackwell.

Marett, V. (1989). *Immigrants Settling in the City*. Leicester: Leicester University Press.

Market and Opinion Research International (MORI). (1989). *Research on Alternative Medicine*. Cited in S. Cant and U. Sharma, *A New Medical Pluralism? Alternative Medicine, Doctors, Patients and the State.* London: UCL Press.

Marks, L., and Hilder, L. (1997). Ethnic advantage: Infant survival among Jewish and Bengali immigrants in East London 1870–1990. In M. Worboys and L. Marks (Eds.), *Migrants, Minorities and Health: Historical and Contemporary Studies*. London: Routledge.

Martin, E. (1989). *The Woman in the Body: A Cultural Analysis of Reproduction*. Milton Keynes: Open University Press.

Martineau, A., White, M., and Bhopal, R. (1997). No sex differences in immunisation rates of British South Asian children: The effect of migration. *British Medical Journal, 314*, 642.

Mason, J. (1997). *Qualitative Researching*. London: Sage.

Massey, D. (1994). *Space, Place and Gender*. Cambridge: Polity Press.

Mathieson, C. M., and Stam, H. J. (1995). Renegotiating identity: Cancer narratives. *Sociology of Health and Illness, 17*, 283–306.

Matthews, D. A., and Larson, D. B. (1997). Faith and medicine: Reconciling the twin traditions of healing. *Mind/Body Medicine, 2*, 3–6.

Meade, M., Horin, J., and Gesler, W. (1988). *Medical Geography.* New York: Guilford Press.

Mechanic, D. (1964). The influence of mothers on their children's health, attitudes and behaviour. *Pediatrics, 33,* 444–453.

Menski, W. (1999). South Asian women in Britain: Family integrity and the primary purpose Rule. In R. Barot, H. Bradley, and S. Fenton (Eds.), *Ethnicity, Gender and Social Change.* Basingstoke: Macmillan.

Miles, A. (1991). *Women, Health and Medicine.* Buckingham-shire: Open University Press.

Modood, T. (1992). *Not Easy Being British: Colour, Culture and Citizenship.* Stoke on Trent: Trentham.

Morley, D., and Robins, K. (1995). *Spaces of Identity: Global Media, Electronic Landscapes and Cultural Boundaries.* London: Routledge.

Mukhi, S.S. (1996). Something to dance about. Retrieved from <http://www.littleindia.com/April96/dance1.html>. Last accessed 1997.

Nagel, J. (1994). Constructing ethnicity: Creating and recreating ethnic identity and culture. *Social Problems, 41,* 152–176.

Narayan, K. (1996). Songs lodged in some hearts: Displacements of women's knowledge in Kangra. In S. Lavie and T. Swedenburg (Eds.), *Displacement, Diaspora and Geographies of Identity.* Durham, NC: Duke University Press.

Nathanson, C. A. (1975). Illness and the feminine role: A theoretical review. *Social Science and Medicine, 9,* 57.

Nathanson, C. A. (1977). Sex, illness and medical care: A review of data, theory and method. *Social Science and Medicine, 11,* 13.

Nazroo, J. (1997). *Ethnicity and Mental Health: Findings from a National Community Survey.* London: Policy Studies Institute.

Nazroo, J., Edwards, A., and Brown, G. (1998). Gender differences in the prevalence of depression: Artefact, alternative disorders, biology or roles? *Sociology of Health and Illness, 20,* 312–330.

Nettleton, S. (1995). *The Sociology of Health and Illness.* Cambridge: Polity Press.

Noerager Stern, P. (Ed.). 1986. *Women, Health and Culture.* Washington, DC: Hemisphere.

Oakley, A. (1980). *Women Confined: Towards a Sociology of Childbirth.* London: Martin Robertson.

Oakley, A. (1981). Interviewing women: A contradiction in terms. In H. Roberts (Ed.), *Doing Feminist Research.* London: Routledge.

Oakley, A. (1986). *From Here to Maternity* (reprint with new introduction). Suffolk: Pelican Books.

Parker, D. (1995). *Through Different Eyes: The Cultural Identities of Young Chinese People in Britain.* Aldershot: Avebury.

Parsons, T. (1951). *The Social System.* New York: Free Press.

Pilgrim, D., and Rogers, A. (1993). *A Sociology of Mental Health and Illness.* Buckinghamshire: Open University Press.

Pill, R., and Stott, W. (1982). Concepts of illness, causation and responsibility: Some preliminary data from a sample of working class mothers. *Social Science and Medicine, 16,* 43–52.

Pitchumon, C. S., and Saran, P. (1976). Health and medical care of Indian immigrants in the United States. In E. Eames and P. Saran (Eds.), *New Ethnics.* New York: Praeger.

Popay, J. (1992). "My health is all right, but I'm just tired all the time": Women's experience of ill health. In H. Roberts (Ed.), *Women's Health Matters.* London: Routledge.

Popay, J., and Groves, A. (2000). "Narrative" in research on gender inequalities in health. In E. Annandale and K. Hunt (Eds.), *Gender Inequalities and Health.* Buckinghamshire: Open University Press.

Popay, J., and Jones, G. (1990). Patterns of health and illness amongst lone parents. *Journal of Social Policy, 19,* 499–534.

Porter, R., and Hinnells, J. R. (Eds.). (1999). *Religion, Health and Suffering.* London: Kegan Paul.

Poster, M. (1984). *Foucault, Marxism and History: Mode of Production versus Mode of Information.* Cambridge: Polity Press.

Pound, P., Gompertz, T., and Ebrahim, S. (1998). Illness in the context of older age: The case of stroke. *Sociology of Health and Illness, 20,* 489–506.

Price, S., and Parr, P. (1996). *Aromatherapy for Babies and Children: Gentle Treatments for Health and Well-Being.* London: Thorsons.

Rack, P. (1982). *Race, Culture and Mental Disorder.* London: Tavistock.

Radley, A., and Billig, M. (1996). Accounts of health and illness: Dilemmas and representations. *Sociology of Health and Illness, 18,* 220–240.

Radley, A., and Green, R. (1987). Chronic illness as adjustment: A methodology and conceptual framework. *Sociology of Health and Illness, 9,* 179–207.

Raftos, M., Mannix, J., and Jackson, D. (1997). More than motherhood? A feminist exploration of women's health in papers indexed by CINAHL (Cumulative Index of Nursing and Allied Health Literature). *Journal of Advanced Nursing, 26,* 1142–1149.

Rajan, R. S. (1993). *Real and Imagined Women.* London: Routledge.

Ram, M. (1996). Ethnography, ethnicity and work: Unpacking the West Midlands clothing industry. In E. S. Lyon and J. Busfield (Eds.), *Methodological Imaginations.* London: Macmillan.

Reed, K. (1998). Contextualising comparative research: The health beliefs and behaviours of American and British South Asian mothers. In S. B. Seperson (Ed.), *Current Proceedings Journal NYSSA (New York State Sociological Association).* New York: New York State Sociological Association.

Reed, K. (2000). Dealing with difference: Researching health beliefs and behaviours of British Asian mothers. *Sociological Research Online, 4* (4). Retrieved from <http://www. socresonline. org.uk/4/4/reed.html>. Last accessed 2001.

Reinharz, S. (1992). *Feminist Research Methods in Social Research.* Oxford: Oxford University Press.

Rhodes, P. J. (1994). Race of interviewer effects: A brief comment. *Sociology, 28,* 547–558.

Roberts, H. (Ed.). (1992). *Women's Health Matters.* London: Routledge.

Rocher, R. (1994). Reconstituting South Asian studies for a diasporic age. Retrieved from <http://asnic.utexas.edu/asnic/sagar/fall.1994/rosane.rocher.art.html>. Last accessed 1997.

Rocheron, Y. (1988). The Asian mother and baby campaign: The construction of ethnic minority health needs. *Critical Social Policy, 22,* 4–23.

Roemer, M. (1977). *Comparative National Policies on Health Care.* New York: Marcel Dekker.

Rosenfeld, S. (1989). The effects of women's employment: personal control and sex differences in mental health. *Journal of Health and Social Behaviour, 30,* 77–91.

Saks, M. (1992). *Alternative Medicine in Britain.* Oxford: Clarendon.

Sargent, C. F., and Johnson, T. M. (Eds.). (1996). *Medical Anthropology: Contemporary Theory and Method.* Westport, CT: Praeger.

Scambler, A., and Scambler, G. (1985). Menstrual symptoms, attitudes and consulting behaviour. *Social Science and Medicine, 20,* 1065–1068.

Scambler, A., and Scambler, G. (1993). *Menstrual Disorder.* London: Routledge.

Schenrich, J. (1987). *Research Methods in the Postmodern*. London: Falmer Press.

Schrijvers, J. (1993). Motherhood experienced and conceptualised: Changing images in Sri Lanka and the Netherlands. In D. Bell, C. Caplan, and W. J. Karim (Eds.), *Gendered Fields: Women, Men and Ethnography*. London: Routledge.

Sharma, U. (1992). *Complementary Medicine Today: Practitioners and Patients*. London: Routledge.

Shilling, C. (1993). *The Body and Social Theory*. London: Sage.

Shotter, J. (1990). Rom Harré: Realism and the turn to social constructionism. In R. Bhaskar (Ed.), *Rom Harré and His Critics*. Oxford: Blackwell.

Showalter, E. (1987). *The Female Malady: Women, Madness and English Culture 1830–1980*. London: Virago.

Singh, P. (1999). Sikh perspectives on health and suffering: A focus on Sikh Theodicy. In J. Hinnells and R. Porter (Eds.), *Religion, Health and Suffering*. London: Kegan Paul.

Skeggs, B. (1997). *Formations of Class and Gender*. London: Sage.

Sloan, R. P, Bagiella, E., and Powell, T. (1999). Religion, spirituality and medicine. *Lancet, 353*, 664–667.

Smith, S. (1993). Residential segregagtion and the politics of racialisation. In M. Cross and M. Keith (Eds.), *Racism, the City and the State*. London: Routledge.

Solomos, J. (1988). *Black youth, Racism and the State*. Cambridge: Cambridge University Press.

Spector, R. (1996). *Cultural Diversity in Health and Illness*. New York: Appleton Century Crofts.

Spivak, G. (1985). Subaltern studies: Deconstructing historiography. In R. Guha (Ed.), *Subaltern Studies: Writings on South Asian History and Society* (vol. 4). London: Oxford University Press.

Stacey, J. (1988). *Brave New Families*. New York: Basic Books.

Stacey, M. (1985). Women and health: The US and the UK compared. In E. Lewin and V. Olesen (Eds.), *Women, Health and Healing: Towards a New Perspective*. New York: Tavistock.

Stones, R. (1996). *Sociological Reasoning: Towards a Past-Modern Sociology*. Basingstoke: Macmillan.

Thomas, R. (1989). Editorial comment. *Journal of Alternative and Complementary Medicine, 7* (6), 5.

Thorogood, N. (1990). Caribbean home remedies and their importance for black women's health in contemporary Britain. In

P. Abbott and G. Payne (Eds.), *New Directions in the Sociology of Health.* London: Falmer Press.

Tong, R. (1992). *Feminist Thought.* London: Routledge.

Trinh, T. M. (1988). "Not you/like you": Post-colonial women and the interlocking questions of identity and difference. Feminism and the critique of colonial discourse [Special issue]. *Inscriptions, 3* (4).

Trinh, T. M. (1989). *Woman, Native, Other.* Bloomington: Indiana University Press.

Turner, B. (1987). *Medical Power and Social Knowledge.* London: Sage.

Turner, B. (1991). Recent developments in the theory of the body. In M. Featherstone, M. Hepworth, and B. Turner (Eds.), *The Body: Social Processes and Cultural Theory.* London: Sage.

Turner, B. (1992). *Regulating Bodies: Essays in Medical Sociology.* London: Routledge.

Turner, R. (1989). Deconstructing the field. In D. Silverman and F. Gubrium (Eds.), *Politics of Field Research: Sociology beyond Enlightenment.* London: Sage.

Visweswaran, K. (1994). *Fictions of Feminist Ethnography.* Minneapolis: University of Minnesota Press.

Watson, J. L. (1977). *Between Two Cultures.* Oxford: Basil Blackwell.

Werbner, P., and Modood, T. (1997). *Debating Cultural Hybridity: Multi-Cultural Identities and the Politics of Anti-Racism.* London: Zed Books.

West, R. (1992). Alternative medicine: Prospects and speculations. In M. Saks (Ed.), *Alternative Medicine in Britain.* Oxford: Clarendon Press.

Williams, R., and Shams, M. (1998). Generational continuity and change in British Asian health and health behaviour. *Journal of Epidemology and Community Health, 52,* 558–563.

Williams, S. J. (1984). The genesis of chronic illness: Narrative reconstruction. *Sociology of Health and Illness, 6,* 175–200.

Williams, S. J. (1996). The vicissitudes of embodiment across the chronic illness trajectory. *Body and Society, 2* (2), 23–47.

Williams, S. J. (2000). Chronic illness as biographical disruption or biographical disruption as chronic illness? Reflections on a core concept. *Sociology of Health and Illness, 22,* 50–67.

Woollett, A., and Dosanjh-Matwala, N. (1990). Pregnancy and antenatal care: The attitudes and experiences of Asian women. *Child: Health Care and Development, 16,* 63–78.

Woollett, A., and Marshall, H. (1997). Discourses of pregnancy and childbirth. In L. Yardley (Ed.), *Material Discourses of Health and Illness*. London: Routledge.

Woollett, A., Marshall, H., Nicolson, P., and Dosanjh-Matwala, N. (1994). Asian women's ethnic identity: The impact of gender and context in the accounts of women bringing up children in East London. In K. K. Bhavani and A. Phoenix (Eds.), *Shifting Identities, Shifting Racisms: A Feminism and Psychology Reader*. London: Sage.

Worsley, P. (1997). *Knowledges: What Different People Make of the World*. London: Profile Books.

Yardley, L. (1997). Introducing material-discursive approaches to health and illness. In L. Yardley (Ed.), *Material Discourses of Health*. London: Routledge.

Index

ABOUT THE AUTHOR

Kate Reed is a lecturer in Sociology at the University of Kent, Canterbury, United Kingdom. Her research interests include sociological theory, health and illness, race and ethnicity, and gender studies.